Blood and Marrow Transplantation

BLOOD AND MARROW TRANSPLANTATION

A Patient's Guide to
Hematopoietic Stem Cell Transplantation

The Blood and Marrow Transplant Program
at the University of Minnesota Medical Center, Fairview

Fairview Press • Minneapolis

Library of Congress Cataloging-in-Publication Data
Blood and marrow transplantation: a patient's guide to hematopoietic stem cell transplantation / Fairview-University Blood and Marrow Transplant Services, affiliated with the University of Minnesota.
     p. cm.
     Includes index
     ISBN 1-57749-114-9 (pb : alk. paper)
     1. Bone marrow--Transplantation--Popular works. 2. Hematopoietic stem cells--Transplantation--Popular works. I. Fairview-University Blood and Marrow Transplant Services.
     RD123.5.B565 2004
     617.4'4--dc21   2001055633

First Printing: August 2004
Printed in the United States of America
08   07   06   05   5   4   3   2

Writer: Linda Picone
General editors: Cynthia Hibbs, RN, PNP, and Leslie Parran, MS, RN, AOCN
Editor: Lee Engfer
Cover designer: *Laurie Ingram Design*
Interior designers: Jane Nicolo and Tim Larson
Illustrations: Barbara Beshoar and Jane Nicolo

"Adult Preparation Checklist: Getting Ready for Transplant" (page 113), "Pediatric Preparation Checklist: Getting Ready for Transplant" (page 121), and "Getting Ready to Leave the Transplant Center: Frequently Asked Questions" (page 127) adapted from materials developed by Caroline Gale, LICSW; Doris Knettel, LICSW; Stacy Stickney Ferguson, LICSW; Janet Ziegler, LICSW; University of Minnesota Medical Center, Fairview, BMT Social Workers; and Kate Montgomery, LICSW, at the Office of Patient Advocacy at the National Marrow Donor Program.

To order additional copies of this book or a free catalog of Fairview Press titles, call toll-free 1-800-544-8207. Or visit our Web site at www.fairviewpress.org. Save 40% when you order 25 or more copies.

This book is dedicated in memory of two individuals who significantly shaped the Blood and Marrow Transplant Program at the University of Minnesota Medical Center, Fairview:

Marline Jensen, who provided over twenty-six years of service as unit secretary. She was loved and appreciated by all our pediatric BMT families as she watched over their children who were receiving BMT.

Bryan Clemens, RN, who in his tenure as staff nurse at the BMT pediatric unit provided excellent nursing care and a wonderful sense of humor, which created a positive environment for pediatric patients and families.

This book is also dedicated to all our patients and their families. You've impressed us with your strength, inspired us with your courage, and honored us with your trust.

ACKNOWLEDGMENTS

Fairview Health Services is a community-focused health system providing a complete range of services, from prevention of illness and injury to care for the most complex medical conditions. The information contained in this book was assembled and developed by the Blood and Marrow Transplant (BMT) Program at the University of Minnesota Medical Center, Fairview.

Primary contributors to this book were Cynthia Hibbs, RN, PNP, and Leslie Parran, MS, RN, AOCN. Many other individuals made significant contributions to this book, including Stacy Stickney Ferguson, MSW, LICSW; Janet Ziegler, MSW, LICSW; Caroline Gale, MSW, LICSW; Doris Knettel, MSW, LICSW; Joanne Howard, RN; Norma Ramsay, MD; and Daniel Weisdorf, MD.

CONTENTS

PREFACE

This book is written for people who will undergo blood or marrow transplant (BMT) using hematopoietic stem cells. Terms such as *allogeneic, matched unrelated donor (MUD), unrelated donor (URD), autologous,* or *cord blood transplant* may also be used when referring to this treatment. This book will help explain the medical procedure and treatment course, providing useful information for:

- Patients who are going to have a BMT

- Caregivers, parents, family members, and friends who are supporting a loved one during such treatment

- Donors who want information about their role and how BMT works

HOW TO USE THIS BOOK

This book will provide information about medical and emotional aspects of BMT. BMT is used to treat many types of cancer, blood disorders, and inherited metabolic diseases.

There are two types of BMT: allogeneic and autologous. Allogeneic transplant is the transfer of stem cells from a donor's blood, bone marrow, or umbilical cord blood to a patient. In autologous transplant, the patient donates and receives back his or her own stem cells.

Allogeneic   Autologous

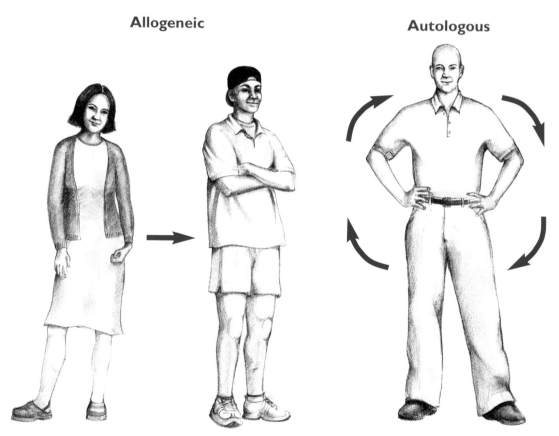

In an allogeneic transplant, a donor's blood, bone marrow, or umbilical cord blood is used as a source of stem cells. An autologous transplant uses stem cells from the patient having the transplant.

While there are similarities between the two types of transplant, aspects of treatment and recovery are different. No matter which type of transplant is recommended, this book offers useful information to all patients, their loved ones, and caregivers.

YOUR ROLE AS PATIENT

Throughout the BMT process, you will work closely with members of your healthcare team. You will rely on the expertise of physicians and other healthcare providers for recommendations and guidance. Patients, parents/guardians of pediatric patients, and significant others are essential members of the healthcare team, too. As a team member, it is important to understand what is happening and what the options are so you can actively take part in decision making. The following are ways to fully participate in your treatment:

How can I participate in my treatment?

- **Learn about your illness and BMT.** Talk to doctors, visit transplant centers, and contact other people who have had a BMT.

- **Search the Internet.** Look at Web sites specific to your disease (see Resources on page 147) as well as general BMT Web sites, including:

    http://www.fairviewbmt.org
    http://www.cancer.umn.edu
    http://www.peds.umn.edu/centers/bmt

- **Refer to Resources** (page 147) for phone numbers, addresses, and Web sites of helpful organizations, including those referenced in this book.

- **Refer to the Preparation Checklists** (appendix A and B).

- **Keep a notebook or journal to organize and manage information.** Write down any questions that you want to ask your doctor, and record the answers that you receive.

- **Ask questions when you don't understand something.** You may need to have information repeated or reworded. Consider recording meetings with your doctor, so you can play and replay the conversation to refresh your memory. Bring someone with you to meetings who can listen and take notes for you.

- **Learn about all the options for your treatment.**

- **Follow through on your treatment plan and any lifestyle changes that are recommended** (for example, quit smoking, limit alcohol consumption, and, if advised, complete necessary dental treatments prior to transplant).

- **Complete daily personal care.** During BMT, this will include mouth care, hygiene, central venous catheter care, nutrition, exercise, leisure activities, and getting dressed in your own clothing.

The BMT Program at the University of Minnesota Medical Center, Fairview

From the world's first successful transplant in 1968 to the establishment of our BMT program in 1974, the Blood and Marrow Transplant Program at the University of Minnesota Medical Center, Fairview, has developed into a world-class program with a reputation for innovation and excellence in BMT. We use a family-centered, interdisciplinary approach to care for people receiving hematopoietic stem cell transplants. Our mission at the Blood and Marrow Transplant Program is to continue this legacy through unity in our commitment to provide expert, excellent, and innovative care to blood and marrow transplant patients and families throughout the continuum of their care experience. Our staff coordinates referrals and many aspects of patient care. After referral to the University of Minnesota Medical Center, Fairview, the staff will:

- Coordinate communication between you, your referring physician, the BMT physicians and nurses, and other hospital departments.

- Work with the hospital's patient financial services representatives and your insurance company regarding insurance coverage.

- Communicate with you and your referring physician about your medical condition and possible dates for evaluation and admission.

To contact us for referral or information regarding the BMT Program, University of Minnesota Medical Center, Fairview, call toll free 1-888-601-0787, or, within the Minneapolis-St. Paul area, 612-273-2800.

Here are some milestones in the history of our program:

1968: World's first successful human bone marrow transplant, performed by University of Minnesota physicians in an infant with an immune deficiency syndrome.

1974: BMT program established at the University of Minnesota as an independent program to treat pediatric patients.

1975: First successful transplant in a patient with lymphoma.

1979: Adult BMT program established and joint BMT program formed with pediatrics.

1982: First transplant for inherited metabolic disease.

1985: One of the first BMTs using an unrelated donor is performed.

1980s: Development of autologous marrow transplantation—using the patient's own marrow—for chronic myelogenous leukemia.

1991: First cord blood transplant performed with a related donor for a child with leukemia.

1992: Began using autologous BMT to treat breast cancer.

1996: University of Minnesota Cancer Research Center opens, providing contiguous lab space for both pediatric and adult BMT researchers.

1998: University of Minnesota Cancer Center, affiliated with Fairview-University BMT Services, becomes a National Cancer Institute designated "Comprehensive Cancer Center."

1998: The 30th anniversary of the program.

1999: The 3000th transplant performed.

1999: The first sickle cell patient receiving a non-myeloablative allogeneic sibling donor transplant.

1999: The American Red Cross, Fairview-University Medical Center, and the University of Minnesota team up to open the Midwest's first public cord blood bank.

2000: The world's first cord blood transplant is performed on a patient with Fanconi anemia using pre-implantation genetic testing to ensure the donor's umbilical cord blood would provide a perfect tissue match.

2000: The first successful double-cord blood transplant for the BMT program.

2001: Non-myeloablative transplantation is performed using sibling, unrelated, or cord blood sources.

2003: The 4000th transplant performed.

2004: Successful early experience of leukemia reinduction using immunoablative therapy along with haploidentical donor natural killer cells.

2004: Published high success rates in recipients of umbilical cord blood transplantation after nonmyeloablative therapy in older adults (over 45 years old).

PATIENT FINANCIAL SERVICES

Patient financial services representatives will work with you, your insurance company, and your physician to arrange for payment for transplant-related services. Patient financial services is also available to discuss payment options.

THE HEALTHCARE TEAM

The BMT Program uses a team approach to provide high-quality, compassionate care.

Each member of your healthcare team is experienced in blood and marrow transplant. Team members meet regularly to talk about patient care and coordinate decisions with patients about what happens during their BMT.

BMT Nurse Coordinators

BMT nurse coordinators will be involved throughout your pre-transplant evaluation, hospital stay, recovery, discharge, and outpatient care. They are available to:

- Discuss your disease, the purpose of BMT, the pre-transplant process, the transplant, and possible complications.

- Relate key information about expected workup dates, transplant dates, and finding a suitable donor (if needed).

- Work with the BMT physicians to coordinate patient care, testing, and treatment planning.

- Coordinate your plan of care with other members of the healthcare team on an inpatient and outpatient basis.

- Communicate with referring physicians.

- Prepare you to leave the transplant center and return home.

Medical Staff

Physicians, Nurse Practitioners, and Physician Assistants

The physicians in the BMT Program include:

- **Attending physicians**—specialists in blood and marrow transplantation. Some attending physicians treat adult patients, while others work with pediatric patients (children). They are the most knowledgeable and experienced persons on the transplant team. They will be in charge of your overall treatment plan.

- **Consultants**—experts in medical subspecialty areas such as lung (pulmonary), infectious, or kidney disease. They may be called for advice and consultation about your treatment.

- **Medical fellows**—pediatricians or internal medicine specialists who are getting additional training in blood and marrow transplantation, hematology, and oncology.

- **Residents**—physicians taking advanced training to become pediatricians or internal medicine specialists.

Nurse practitioners (NPs) and physician assistants (PAs) can prescribe medication and treatment. They work closely with the attending physicians.

An attending physician, medical fellow, resident, physician assistant, or nurse practitioner will see you daily while you are in the hospital. The attending physician makes daily rounds and is available twenty-four hours a day. Attending physicians on the inpatient unit change periodically, but all patients have a primary attending physician who will see them in follow-up visits after they leave the hospital.

Consultant physicians from subspecialties may be asked to see you about a specific concern or treatment, but the attending transplant physician will be in charge of your care.

All the physicians who see you during treatment will meet regularly to discuss your plan of care. You, your family members, and your significant other can address questions or concerns with any member of the medical team.

Nursing Staff

Nurses working on the BMT unit and in the BMT clinic are specially trained to care for BMT patients. On the inpatient unit, each patient has one primary nurse and several associate nurses. This nursing team oversees your care plan and is available to address questions and concerns.

A charge nurse is responsible for each nursing shift. The charge nurse assigns nurses and nursing assistants to each patient. He or she periodically checks with nurses and patients about patient care and can help answer questions and address concerns.

Your Nursing Care

The primary nursing team members are a link between your family and other nurses and physicians. To benefit the most from your nursing care:

- Participate in planning your care with nursing staff.

- Ask questions

- Share important information (about yourself and family) that can help with treatment

- Learn what care is needed and participate in that care.

Nursing assistants support the nurses by taking vital signs, helping with patient care, and providing for patient comfort needs in the hospital.

Nurses will:

- Routinely assess your vital signs and condition.

- Administer medications, blood products, IV fluids, and the hematopoietic stem cells (transplant).

- Draw blood from your central venous catheter for lab tests.

- Develop a plan of care with you and your healthcare team.

- Educate you and your family throughout the transplant process.

- Help you and your family address psychological support needs.

SUPPORT SERVICES

In addition to the medical and nursing teams, support staff and other services are available to help you before, during, and after the transplant.

Clinical Social Workers

The BMT Program is staffed by social workers who work exclusively with BMT patients and their families. A BMT social worker will contact you and your family before you come for your pre-transplant workup. He or she will help you prepare for the upcoming transplant by addressing practical issues, such as transportation and housing, as well as the emotional impact of having a transplant. A BMT social worker will also meet with you and your family during the pre-transplant workup to assess your needs. During the transplant hospitalization and following discharge, social workers are excellent resources who provide counseling and address specific concerns or problems. They are available to:

- **Answer questions** about housing, transportation, childcare, school, community resources, and insurance.

- **Provide counseling** to individuals, couples, and families who are experiencing emotional stress; teach relaxation techniques; and promote emotional adaptation to illness and treatment.

- **Help with problem solving,** advocacy, and communication about your plan of care.

- **Lead various support groups** that provide patients, caregivers, and family members with information and opportunities to share their experiences.

Child Family Life Specialists

Child family life (CFL) specialists provide age-appropriate opportunities for pediatric patients to express their feelings about their illness and to understand and cope with what is happening to them during their hospitalization and clinic visits. CFL specialists support pediatric patients, their parents, and family members throughout the treatment experience. CFL services may include:

- Pre-admission programs and tours

- Education and preparation for medical procedures

- Support for pediatric patients during medical procedures

- Medical and therapeutic play

- One-to-one bedside visits

- Parent social programs and lunch outings

- Special programs for pediatric patients and siblings

- Interactive children's television shows

- Opportunities to meet celebrities

Spiritual Care and Healing

Facing a disease and choosing to have a BMT is a demanding process—physically, emotionally, and spiritually. It is a life-changing experience for you and for your family. The journey through sickness to healing and well-being is very challenging.

Through interfaith ministry to patients, families, and staff, our chaplains are dedicated to helping patients sustain and deepen their relationships with the sacred and with other people.

The chaplains regard patient and family cultures, beliefs, value systems, and spiritual and faith practices as important resources for healing and well-being. During times of stress, crisis, and life-threatening illness, there may be moments when patients and loved ones are seeking the sacred—trying to find meaning, hope, and peace in new or familiar ways. Our chaplains offer:

- A listening and caring presence

- Spiritual and emotional support and counsel

- Prayer, blessing services, rituals, worship experiences, and sacraments

- Assistance in ethical decision making

- Inspirational and educational resources

- Coordination with leaders of various faith communities

- Complementary therapies (like Healing Touch and meditation)

School

A visiting teacher is available for patients in grades K–12 to help them keep up with their schoolwork. Children are encouraged to use materials and lesson plans from their own schools, but if this isn't possible, hospital teachers will provide materials. For more information, contact your social worker.

Dietitian

A dietitian can answer questions about nutrition and food requests while you're in the hospital and after you go home. If you would like to talk to a dietitian, ask your nurse or doctor to arrange a meeting.

Physical, Occupational, and Speech Therapy

Many BMT patients benefit from working with a physical, occupational, or speech therapist during and after their hospital stay. Working with a physical therapist can be a valuable and vital aspect of recovery. Nurses and physicians help determine whether this therapy is needed.

Care Partners

Care Partners provides nonmedical support services to BMT patients and their families. Volunteers can help in a variety of ways, such as picking up relatives at the airport, playing with or caring for children, helping with errands, shopping, or spending time with the patient.

As part of the Care Partners program, Project IsoLink allows hospitalized patients and their families to keep in touch with friends and family members through the use of computers and free Internet and e-mail access.

Shortly after your arrival in Minneapolis, you will be introduced to the Care Partners program. Care Partners staff will meet with you to identify your needs and provide information on how the program can help you during your transplant stay.

Patients and family members who have used the Care Partners program find the comfort, strength, companionship, and friendship of the volunteers very supportive.

Home Healthcare Services

After being discharged from the hospital, you may need to have a nurse come to your home or temporary residence to answer questions or establish care routines. Some patients, for example, receive IV medications after they leave the hospital, which may require the assistance of a home care nurse.

Home care services that may be provided include:

- Assistance with the administration of medications

- Transfusion of blood products

- Pain management

- IV nutrition or tube feedings

- Drawing blood or obtaining samples for lab tests, then monitoring test results

LIFE ON THE BMT INPATIENT UNIT

Regular Nursing Care

Nurses take patient vital signs—blood pressure, pulse rate, respiratory rate, and temperature. They check vital signs every four hours.

The schedule for checking vital signs is usually 8 A.M., 12 P.M., 4 P.M., 8 P.M., 12 A.M., and 4 A.M. The nursing staff may check vital signs more frequently if your condition changes or if certain medications or transfusions of blood products are given.

Early each morning, between 4 and 6 A.M., nurses draw blood from each patient's central venous catheter. Blood is rarely drawn from the arm. Blood tests help determine and guide patient care for the day.

Nurses measure patients' fluid intake and output. Patients are asked to save all urine and stool samples in their bathrooms and to report the amounts of fluid they drink.

Mouth care is usually performed four times each day. This includes cleaning your teeth with toothettes (small sponges) soaked in a salt (saline) solution. You should also clean your gum lines, tongue, and cheek pouches and rinse your mouth with the solution, spitting after each rinse.

Patients are weighed every morning between 7 and 9 A.M., sometimes twice a day if there is any concern that a patient is gaining or losing too much weight or fluids.

Central venous catheter dressings are changed daily or as needed based on the type of dressing, how well the dressing is staying on, dressing cleanliness, and whether the dressing is wet or moist.

Intensive Nursing Care

The BMT unit also provides care to patients who become critically ill and require ventilator or other intensive care support. When patients require more intensive nursing care, nurses provide more continuous care and monitoring.

Because intensive care requires increased assessment, observation, and patient monitoring, patient rooms may seem less private and more busy. It may be more difficult for family members to rest in patient rooms. Nursing staff will work with families to promote optimal patient care and family visitation.

Daily Routine

Meals are served at about 8 A.M., 12 P.M., and 5 P.M. each day. Patients receive a menu daily and choose meals for the next day. Dietary staff members are available to help with menu selections.

Adult patients and older children take a shower every day to reduce the risk of infection. Small children are given a daily bath.

Physical activity is important to prevent weakness and lung complications. Patients are encouraged to do some physical activity in their rooms each day to maintain strength and endurance. Exercise bikes and other equipment are available for patient use.

Patients are also encouraged to dress in comfortable clothing while in the hospital. Many patients say they feel better psychologically when they are up and dressed every day.

Visitors are important to patients but are limited to no more than three at a time in the patient's hospital room. This is necessary to support optimal air quality.

Infection Control

When undergoing BMT, patients are at higher risk of infection. To reduce the chance of infection on the unit:

- Anyone entering a patient's room must wash his or her hands with an antiseptic soap for fifteen seconds or use a rinseless degermer (waterless soap).

- Children under age sixteen must have an Infectious Disease Screening Form completed for them before entering a patient's room.

- Hospital staff or visitors with signs of a cold must wear a mask at all times on the unit.

- The doors to patients' rooms will be kept closed. If a door is held open for more than thirty seconds, an alarm will go off, indicating that the door should be closed to permit continuous air filtration.

- No plants—not even dried—are allowed in patients' rooms. Silk flowers are allowed, but any moss at the base of flower arrangements must be removed. Although flowers are a traditional gift, plants and the dirt they are potted in can carry molds or fungi that are harmful to people recovering from BMT.

BMT CLINIC

Patients are discharged from the hospital as soon as their treatment and condition can be supported on an outpatient basis. Patient care is then managed at our BMT clinic.

The BMT clinic provides care every day of the year to transplant patients in various phases of treatment: pre-transplant, transplant, and post-transplant, including transplant anniversary visits. Care includes provider visits (physicians, nurse practitioners, or physician assistants), laboratory tests, IV fluids, IV antibiotics, electrolyte replacement, blood products, chemotherapy, and stem cell reinfusions. Some diagnostic procedures are also performed at the clinic, including bone marrow biopsies, skin biopsies, and spinal taps for older children and adults.

Understanding Blood or Marrow Transplant (BMT)

CHAPTER ONE

This chapter provides a basic overview of blood and bone marrow transplantation.

You'll read about:

The history of bone marrow transplantation

Stem cells and the immune system

How BMT works

When BMT may help

THE HISTORY OF BONE MARROW TRANSPLANTATION

The first successful bone marrow transplant was performed in an infant with an immune deficiency at the University of Minnesota Hospital, now the University of Minnesota Medical Center, Fairview, in 1968. Doctors replaced the baby's unhealthy bone marrow with marrow donated from his sister. The new marrow repaired the baby's defective immune system and the baby grew into a healthy adult.

The first autologous transplants, which use a patient's own bone marrow, were performed in the early 1980s. Transplants using marrow from unrelated donors began in the mid-1980s. In the early 1990s, stem cells collected from circulating blood began to be used in transplants, first autologous and then, more recently, from donors. Umbilical cord blood was also used as a new source of donor stem cells in the early 1990s.

Why are bone marrow transplants used?

At first, transplants were used as part of treatment for aplastic anemia and immune deficiencies. The transplants replaced missing or defective marrow, blood, and immune cells. Later, bone marrow transplants were used to treat leukemias or cancers of the bone marrow. Since then, the procedure has been expanded to treat many other conditions, including diseases that don't involve the bone marrow. Today, doctors are using stem cell transplants to treat specific blood disorders, metabolic diseases, immunological diseases, and many kinds of cancer.

Researchers have developed better methods for matching donors with patients and improved drugs for preventing rejection of the new stem cells. These advances have allowed patients to leave the hospital earlier and continue their treatment on an outpatient basis.

STEM CELLS AND THE IMMUNE SYSTEM

Bone marrow is the spongy tissue inside your bones where blood cells are made. The "parent cells" of all blood cells are called *hematopoietic stem cells*. Stem cells divide and form the different cells that make up your blood and your immune system. Stem cells make millions of blood cells every day. The three main types of blood cells are:

What are stem cells?

Red blood cells. These cells form the "blood" we're most familiar with. Red blood cells travel from the heart and lungs, carrying oxygen to the rest of your body. The oxygen is carried on molecules called *hemoglobin*. Most of your blood cells are red blood cells. A low number of red cells (or low hemoglobin) can make you tired or breathless.

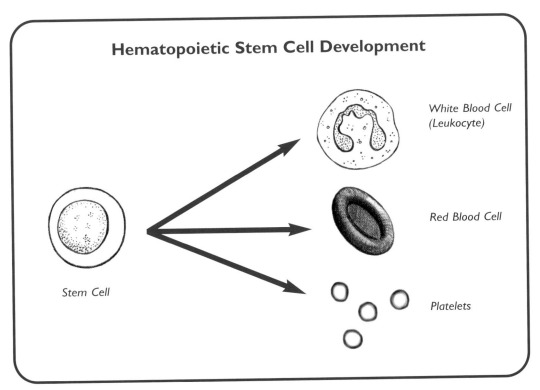

Hematopoietic Stem Cell Development

White Blood Cell (Leukocyte)

Red Blood Cell

Platelets

Stem Cell

Stem cells divide and mature to produce white blood cells (leukocytes), red blood cells, and platelets.

White blood cells. White blood cells fight infection and, therefore, are an important part of the immune system. A low white blood cell count increases the risk of developing an infection. There are several kinds of white blood cells. *Neutrophils* are important white cells that help fight infections caused by bacteria and yeasts. Others, called *lymphocytes,* carry the immunologic memory to protect against viral and other infections, especially those for which people receive vaccinations.

Platelets. Platelets help your blood to clot when you have an injury. They are smaller than red and white blood cells. A low platelet count increases the risk of bleeding and bruising.

HOW BMT WORKS

To prepare for BMT, high doses of drugs (called *chemotherapy*) and sometimes radiation are given for two reasons: to destroy cancer or disease and to suppress the patient's immune system, preventing rejection of the transplant. An intravenous infusion (transplant) of stem cells, previously donated by you or by a donor, should restore your ability to make blood cells. These stem cells plant themselves in your bone marrow, almost like seeds in the ground, and reproduce, making new bone marrow and new blood cells.

How does
BMT work?

The term *BMT* is a bit confusing. It sounds like an operation, like an organ transplant, but it is not a surgical procedure. It's more like a blood transfusion. You may wonder, too, what the difference is between bone marrow transplant, peripheral blood stem cell transplant, and umbilical cord blood transplant. The main difference is the source of the stem cells and how they are collected. Regardless of their source, stem cells are given to the patient in the same way: by intravenous (IV) infusion.

Transplant Cell Sources: Bone Marrow, Peripheral Blood, Umbilical Cord Blood

In a bone marrow transplant, hematopoietic stem cells are collected from your own bone marrow or from a donor's. Bone marrow is aspirated from the pelvic bones using a special needle and syringe.

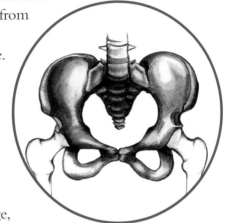

Stem cells can also be collected from blood. These stem cells are referred to as peripheral blood stem cells. They are collected, or "harvested," using a large intravenous (IV) needle or a special IV catheter called a *central venous catheter*. In a peripheral blood stem cell harvest, the blood circulates through a special centrifuge, which removes the white blood cells along with the stem cells and then returns the red blood cells to the body. This procedure is often referred to as *apheresis* or, more specifically, *leukapheresis*. It is done on an outpatient basis.

Bone marrow, which contains stem cells, is found throughout the body. For a bone marrow transplant, marrow is collected from the pelvic bones in a minor surgical procedure.

A third source of stem cells is blood from the umbilical cord and placenta of a newborn. This blood is a particularly rich source of stem cells, taken from what is normally discarded after a baby is delivered. Cord blood from a related or unrelated baby donor may be used for transplant. Some hospitals collect cord blood (with parental consent) for donation to cord blood banks.

In this book, the term *BMT* is used for any transplant involving stem cells, regardless of their source.

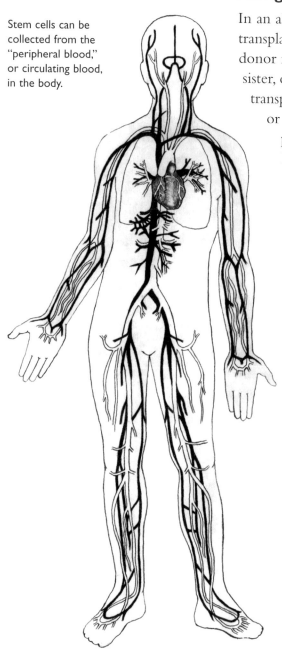

Stem cells can be collected from the "peripheral blood," or circulating blood, in the body.

Transplant Types: Allogeneic and Autologous

In an allogeneic BMT (sometimes called *allo* transplant), stem cells come from a donor. The donor may be a relative, usually a brother or sister, or an unrelated donor. Unrelated donor transplants are sometimes referred to as URD or MUD (matched unrelated donor) transplants. To find a suitable donor, you'll have your blood tested and typed so that it can be compared to blood samples of potential donors. This typing, called *HLA typing,* is a way to find a donor who is a good match for you so that your body won't reject the transplanted stem cells.

An autologous BMT (sometimes called *auto* transplant) uses stem cells taken from your own body. Drugs called *growth factors,* which encourage the growth of stem cells, are given prior to harvesting the stem cells. Stem cells are then collected from your blood or bone marrow and are processed, frozen, and stored. After your treatment with chemotherapy and/or radiation, the harvested cells are thawed and transfused back into your bloodstream through the central venous catheter.

The type of transplant selected depends on your disease, your age, and whether a donor is available. Most people with leukemia have an allogeneic transplant, for example, while those with a solid tumor or a lymphoma are more likely to have an autologous transplant.

WHEN BMT MAY HELP

The number of diseases for which BMT may be recommended is growing. For some diseases, such as leukemia, BMT is used to replace unhealthy or cancerous bone marrow. For other diseases, such as Hodgkin's disease, the bone marrow may be healthy, but BMT replaces stem cells that are destroyed during high-dose chemotherapy and radiation treatments used to eliminate the disease. For patients with inherited diseases, BMT provides missing enzymes or cells.

When is BMT helpful?

Diseases and Conditions for which BMT May Be Used

Leukemia

Acute Lymphocytic Leukemia (ALL)

Acute Myelogenous Leukemia (AML)

Chronic Lymphocytic Leukemia (CLL)

Chronic Myelogenous Leukemia (CML)

Juvenile Myelomonocytic Leukemia (JMML)

Lymphoma

Hodgkin's Disease   Non-Hodgkin's Lymphoma

Solid Tumors

Ewing's Sarcoma   Neuroblastoma

Renal Cell Cancer   Brain Tumors

Multiple Myeloma

Myelodysplastic Syndrome (MDS)

Inherited Metabolic Disorders

Adrenoleukodystrophy (ALD)

Globoid Cell

Hurler's Syndrome

Maroteaux-Lamy Syndrome

Metachromatic Leukodystrophy (MLD)

Krabbe's Disease

Aplastic Anemia

Immune Deficiency

Other Inherited Disorders

Sickle Cell Anemia   Fanconi Anemia

Osteopetrosis   Thalassemia

CHAPTER TWO

GETTING READY FOR BMT

Planning and preparing for BMT will be stressful for you and your family. This chapter discusses emotional and practical ways to prepare for a transplant, explaining the pre-transplant evaluation and other steps that are taken before the procedure.

In this chapter, you'll read about:

The referral process

Choosing a caregiver

Handling insurance issues and expenses

Preparing emotionally

The pre-transplant evaluation

Getting a central venous catheter

THE REFERRAL PROCESS

How do I know
if I need a BMT?

If your doctor thinks you may benefit from a BMT, he or she will refer you to a stem cell transplant program or center. Before making a decision to go ahead with the transplant, it is important to understand as much as you can. BMT is effective for many people, but it's not a simple procedure, and it may result in permanent life changes. Often, the decision to have a BMT comes at a time when you may already feel overwhelmed both by the disease you have and the treatments you've been through.

Individuals involved in the referral process include:

- Patient/family

- Referring physician

- Attending transplant physician

- Administrative nurse coordinator

- Patient financial representative

- Insurance representative
  (often called a transplant case manager)

- Social worker

When you first meet with doctors and others at the transplant center, you and your family may have many questions. Every question you have is a good question to ask—this is your treatment and you have a right to understand what it involves. You may want to write questions down before meeting with the medical team. It also helps to have a family member or friend with you to take notes and provide support.

Arranging a BMT Consultation/Referral

Consultations and referrals to The Blood and Marrow Transplant Program at the University of Minnesota Medical Center, Fairview, can be made by phoning the administrative nurse coordinators at 612-273-2800 or (toll-free) 888-601-0787, or by faxing 612-273-2919. Please have the following information available when making initial contact for a referral:

- Diagnosis and status of disease

- Demographic information, including insurance information

- A brief, one-page medical summary outlining your medical status and clinical treatment course

Following the initial referral call:

- The BMT program will contact you to schedule a consultation appointment with a BMT physician.

- The BMT physician will follow up with a letter to your referring physician regarding your consultation visit.

- The BMT program will contact your insurance company to begin the financial approval process.

Questions to Ask

Some questions to ask the transplant program staff are:

- Why is BMT being recommended now? Are there other options?

- What kind of BMT will be best for me? What does it involve?

- How am I expected to benefit from BMT? What is my prognosis afterward?

- What are the risks of BMT?

- How will a donor be found, if I need one?

How do I decide whether to have a BMT?

- How long is treatment likely to take? How much of that time will I be in the hospital?

- How long do I need to remain near the BMT clinic and hospital?

- What will my life be like after BMT? What are the short-term and long-term side effects?

- What expenses are there with BMT (physicians, hospital, medications, and so forth)?

- What are my nonmedical expenses (such as housing, travel, and meals)?

- Will my insurance cover BMT? If not, what other options are there to pay for it?

Once you've made the decision to go ahead with BMT, there are a number of steps before the actual procedure. Getting ready for your BMT involves practical matters, such as dealing with insurance issues, as well as medical preparation, which happens during the pre-transplant evaluation. It's also important to take some time to prepare yourself emotionally. Staff members from the BMT program are ready to help you and your family at each stage of the process.

CHOOSING A CAREGIVER

A caregiver is a family member or friend who can be with you for the majority of your BMT treatment and recovery. Caregivers can rotate, but an adult is needed to help you throughout your post-transplant care. As difficult as it may seem to find someone to fill this role, the caregiver is a key component of a full and safe recovery. It's important to start deciding who can fill this role prior to coming to the hospital to begin the "workup" evaluation.

We encourage the caregiver to be present during the workup process, as the medications given during a bone marrow biopsy may cause drowsiness. It is also necessary for a caregiver to be available when your central venous catheter is placed; this is often an outpatient procedure requiring anesthesia. In both cases, your caregiver will need to escort you home.

A caregiver sometimes helps with medical tasks, such as giving medication and identifying symptoms to report to the doctor. Some treatments, such as IV medication and nutritional support, which cannot be completed during the BMT clinic hours, are given at home. Initially, a home care nurse may administer these treatments, though often caregivers or patients are trained to do this. The caregiver's primary function, however, is to support you and help you if you become sick.

Who might make a good caregiver?

Other tasks for caregivers may include: driving or accompanying you to the clinic, preparing meals, overseeing medications, and calling for emergency assistance if you are injured, become ill, or develop a fever. You may be doing some of these tasks on your own; however, most patients initially experience fatigue and lack of concentration after high doses of chemotherapy or radiation.

Having a caregiver present is an essential safety precaution, as patients may have an increased risk of bleeding and infection depending on their blood counts. A caregiver also provides needed emotional support throughout treatment and recovery.

Your choice of caregivers will depend on who is available. Different friends and relatives may have different talents and skills that will be helpful. One relative might be available for emotional support, for example, while a friend who is a good organizer might assist with medical care, finances, or transportation.

Do I really need a caregiver?

It's not always easy to find a caregiver, especially for patients who are very independent, are used to living alone, or do not like to ask for help. But doing it on your own isn't an option. You will need help. If you can't think of someone who could be your caregiver, you may be able to find several support people who can take turns. Often, volunteers from your neighborhood or faith community can help with transportation. Several family members or friends might be able to rotate weeks, taking vacation time to be with you. Maybe a family member who is retired can help.

For more information about caregivers, see chapter 7.

HANDLING INSURANCE ISSUES AND EXPENSES

Most BMTs are covered by insurance. Upon referral, a patient financial representative is assigned to each patient. The patient financial representative identifies sources of payment for the BMT. However, there may be additional expenses related to travel, lodging, meals, parking, and long-distance telephone calls. Moreover, there may be changes to the household income when family members take time off work to be caregivers.

Sometimes insurance will provide reimbursement for nonmedical expenses related to traveling away from home for medical treatment. Often, insurers assign a transplant case manager, who can help you identify what will be covered by insurance and what your financial responsibilities will be. It's important to understand your copay responsibilities and insurance coverage for home healthcare and durable medical equipment.

Whether or not you have private medical coverage, it may be to your benefit to apply for assistance through Supplemental Security Income (SSI), Medicare or Medicaid, and Social Security Disability Insurance (SSDI). If you have private insurance, these programs may provide supplemental benefits to assist you with medical expenses that are not covered by your primary insurance.

The programs that most commonly provide benefits to pediatric BMT patients are SSI and Medicaid. It is important to complete applications for the programs as soon as possible, even if you're not sure you will be eligible for benefits. If you are determined to be eligible, programs will often use the date of application as the date on which benefits begin. Your social worker can assist you in obtaining necessary forms and information.

Will insurance cover all my transplant expenses?

The following are important first steps to take in applying for SSI, Medicare, or Medicaid:

SSI:

- Call or visit your local social security office to initiate an application for SSI.

- Ask your social worker to fax a request for an initial interview.

Medicare or Medicaid:

- Call or visit your local human services, social services, or welfare office (counties use various names to describe the office that administers Medicare and Medicaid).

- Request information about applying for Medicare or Medicaid.

- When making initial contact with the office, ask if assistance (for meals, lodging, and transportation related to medical treatment) will be retroactive to the date of application, should you be eligible for benefits.

Am I eligible for medical assistance?

It is helpful to keep a record of all telephone calls, letters related to assistance programs, medical bills, and receipts. If you receive medical bills while your application for medical assistance is pending, inform the billing party that an application has been made.

The following brief descriptions will help you gain a general understanding of these programs. Please ask your social worker for additional information.

- **SSI** provides financial benefits to blind or disabled adults and children who have limited incomes or resources. It is important to apply for SSI as soon as possible because if you are eligible, benefits go into effect on the first of the month following the month of application (or benefits may be retroactive from the date of approval). Children under eighteen qualify for these benefits if they meet social security's definition of *disability* and if their parents' assets and incomes fall within certain guidelines. Once a child turns eighteen, his or her parents' assets and income are no longer considered.

Are children eligible for medical assistance?

Local social security offices review financial resources in determining financial eligibility for benefits. State offices called Disability Determination Services review medical information to determine if patients meet social security's definition of disability. In general, an individual is considered disabled if he or she has a mental or physical condition that results in marked and severe functional limitations. The condition must last or be expected to last twelve months or must be expected to result in the person's death.

- **SSDI** pays benefits to the disabled person and certain members of his or her family if the "insured" (the disabled person) has worked long enough and paid social security taxes.

    You should apply for SSDI at any social security office or by telephone as soon as you become disabled.

- **Medicaid** is a healthcare program for children and adults with low incomes and limited assets. Federal and state governments jointly finance Medicaid. In most states, those who qualify for SSI also qualify for Medicaid. In some states, Medicaid comes automatically with SSI. In others, you must apply for the programs separately. Some people will be eligible for Medicaid even if they are ineligible for SSI. (A child, for example, may be *medically eligible* for benefits, but his or her parents may have too high an income or too many assets to qualify for SSI).

    If you are eligible for Medicaid, assistance may be retroactive for up to three months from the date of application, so it is important to apply as soon as possible.

• **Medicare** is a federal health insurance program for people ages sixty-five or older and for people who have received social security disability benefits for two years. Most children cannot receive Medicare coverage until they are age twenty. The only exception to this rule is children with chronic renal disease who need either a kidney transplant or maintenance dialysis. Children in these situations can receive Medicare benefits if a parent is either receiving social security or has worked long enough to be covered by social security.

PREPARING EMOTIONALLY

By the time you have to make a decision about BMT, you've already had to cope with the knowledge that you have a life-threatening disease. You may have been through times of encouraging news and frightening news.

Coping with a life-threatening disease and the aggressive treatments needed to fight it requires a great deal of emotional strength. It's also an emotional experience for your caregivers and family members. It is normal for feelings to fluctuate. Sometimes you'll feel able to cope, and other times you'll feel numb or overwhelmed.

Are my mood swings normal?

It's normal to feel anger, fear, anxiety, and depression. You might also feel hopeful and optimistic. It is important to not let negative feelings get in the way of your health and your life. Having a positive attitude can help you get through the process.

The following suggestions may be helpful in preparing emotionally for the transplant.

• **Express your feelings.** For example, if you're feeling anxious, afraid, or resentful, talking to other people about it can help you "process" the feelings. If you don't feel comfortable talking to family or friends, consider talking with a counselor, social worker, or therapist.

- **Seek support from family and friends.** Spend time with people who care about you.

- **Take some time to do the things you most enjoy.** Listen to music you love. Watch your favorite movies again. Treat yourself to a massage or manicure. Read a good book.

How can I prepare myself emotionally?

- **Think about positive memories or times in your life.** Reminisce with family and friends.

- **Live every day to the fullest.** Instead of focusing on why this illness has happened to you, try to enjoy simple pleasures, such as the taste of orange juice in the morning or a hug from a loved one.

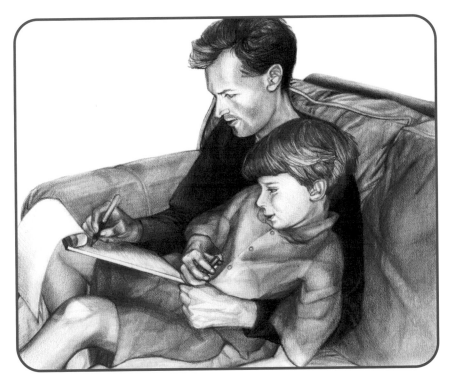

Live each day to the fullest, spending time with the people you love.

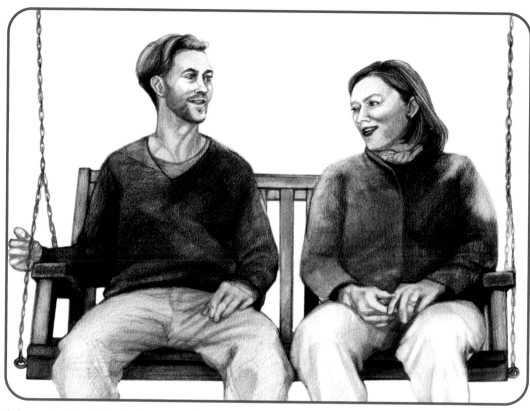

Ask your family and friends for support. Express your feelings, and make plans for when you're feeling better.

- **Get organized.** Some people find it helpful to arrange financial and legal affairs and delegate tasks so they can focus on other things.

- **Pamper yourself.** Pay attention to your own needs—and share them with others. If you need to rest, then rest. If you need a hug, ask for a hug. If you just need someone to listen, find someone who will do that.

- **Get in touch with your spirituality.** Prayer or meditation can be a source of comfort.

- **Find ways to reduce stress.** Learn and use stress reduction techniques such as muscle relaxation, yoga, breathing techniques, imagery, visualization, and meditation. Creative activities such as painting, journal writing, and playing music can also help you deal with stress.

- **Make plans for things you would like to do when you're feeling better.** Plan an event, for example, or find a class you'd like to take.

THE PRE-TRANSPLANT EVALUATION

Before the BMT process begins, you will need to have a medical examination, or workup, to evaluate your eligibility for transplant. The workup will be completed at the outpatient Blood and Marrow Transplant Clinic. When your workup has been scheduled, the social worker will call you and let you know what to expect. During the workup, members of the medical team complete laboratory and diagnostic tests in order to make sure that you are physically ready for the transplant. The workup evaluation takes approximately one week. You should plan on spending six to eight hours each day having diagnostic tests and meeting with healthcare team members. The tests will help physicians evaluate your lung, liver, kidney, and heart function. Overall, the workup provides the medical team with the information necessary to start the transplant process. The evaluation includes:

What happens at the pre-transplant evaluation?

- An in-depth medical history and physical exam

- Blood tests

- Blood, urine, and other cultures

- Kidney function evaluation

- Chest X-rays

- Bone marrow aspiration and biopsy, if there is a possibility that the disease may affect the bone marrow

- Heart evaluation, including an electrocardiogram (ECG or EKG) and an echocardiogram or MUGA scan.

- A spinal tap, if there is a possibility that the disease may affect the spinal fluid

- Consultation with other medical specialties as needed

- Radiation therapy consultation (if needed)

- CT or MRI scans (if needed)

In addition to tests and medical consultations, you'll meet with a physician and nurse coordinator to discuss the BMT process in detail. They'll give you specific information about what you can expect. This is a time to ask more questions about the transplant process. You will also meet with a social worker who will provide information and resources to address your psychosocial needs.

The Pre-Transplant Conference

A pre-transplant conference is a meeting with one of the transplant physicians to discuss your workup evaluation results, decide if BMT is the right treatment for you, and decide on the best timing for the transplant. It is helpful to bring a family member or close friend to this conference to take notes.

Before your treatment can begin, consent forms for treatment need to be discussed and signed. Signing these forms confirms that you understand and are willing to proceed with the transplant therapy. Sometimes you are also asked to participate in research studies, which usually test ways to make transplantation safer and more effective. These studies are optional—you may choose whether or not to participate. If you wish to take part in these studies, you will need to sign additional consent forms. These documents can be overwhelming, since they have to list all the possible risks and complications of BMT. It is important to read consent forms carefully and ask for explanations of anything you don't understand.

For patients under eighteen years old, the parents or legal guardians will sign the consent forms. Children between the ages of eight and seventeen may have their own assent forms to sign. The forms give children an explanation of what will happen to them during the transplant. It is important for children and parents to use this opportunity to talk about the transplant process.

Getting a Central Venous Catheter

At some point during the pre-transplant process, you will have a thin tube called a *central venous catheter* inserted. The catheter makes it possible for the medical team to draw blood; give drugs, fluids, and nutritional supplements; collect stem cells; transfuse blood products; and transfuse the stem cells on your transplant day.

Placement of the catheter is usually done on an outpatient basis in an operating room or radiology procedure room at the hospital. You will be put under local or general anesthesia, and a small incision (about 1 inch) will be made in your neck or below your collarbone. The catheter is put into a large vein leading to your heart. The other end of the catheter is tunneled under the skin and exits through a small incision in your upper chest area. The catheter will be left in throughout the transplant process. You will be taught how to care for the catheter to prevent it from becoming infected or clotted.

What is a central venous catheter?

THE TRANSPLANT PROCESS

This chapter provides an overview of the transplant process, including the different types of transplant, stem cell collection, preparation for transplant, and the transplant procedure.

In this chapter, you'll read about:

Autologous transplants

Allogeneic transplants

Finding a donor

The donation process

Preparing for your transplant

The transplant

Engraftment

AUTOLOGOUS TRANSPLANTS

When your own stem cells are being used for the transplant, you are having an autologous stem cell transplant. Stem cells are collected from your own bone marrow or blood, then they are processed and frozen. After you undergo intensive chemotherapy with or without radiation, the stem cells are then infused (transplanted) back into your body.

For adult patients, much of the autologous stem cell transplant can be done on an outpatient basis. Children may have to stay in the hospital longer.

ALLOGENEIC TRANSPLANTS

A BMT using stem cells from a donor is called an allogeneic transplant. The stem cells may come from a relative or an unrelated donor. They are obtained from the donor's blood or bone marrow or from donated umbilical cord blood.

Related Donors

A related donor transplant can be done if you have a blood relative, usually a brother or sister, whose "tissue type" matches or nearly matches yours. Tissue typing is done through a blood test called the *human leukocyte antigen (HLA) test*. It examines proteins called *antigens* on the surface of white blood cells. Everyone inherits a unique set of these antigens from each parent, sort of like a cellular fingerprint. HLA proteins are markers that help your immune system distinguish "self" (your cells and tissues) from "nonself" (someone else's cells and tissues). Your body can reject cells with different HLA types.

What is tissue typing?

The closer the match between your HLA type and that of the donor, the lower the risk of complications, including rejection and graft-versus-host disease (GVHD), discussed on page 51. Identical twins have identical HLA proteins. Usually the best donor for allo-geneic stem cell transplant is a brother or sister. Siblings have a one-in-four chance of being the same HLA type (matched donor).

Unrelated Donors

If no HLA-matched relative is available, a transplant using stem cells from an unrelated donor may be an option. The donor is a volunteer who has joined a blood and marrow donor registry. In the United States, the National Marrow Donor Program (NMDP) has a registry of millions of potential volunteer donors, with millions of others available through international registries. The donor's stem cells are removed (harvested) on the day of your transplant and then carefully packaged and transported to the transplant facility.

How are donors found?

Umbilical Cord Blood

Stem cells circulate in a baby's blood at the time of birth. These cells can be collected by draining the blood from the umbilical cord and placenta after a baby is delivered. This blood is normally thrown away with the placenta. Cord blood can come from a related baby, but the baby and patient are usually unrelated. Cord blood banks will HLA-type, freeze, and store this blood. If an HLA match is close enough, these cord blood cells can be used for BMT.

FINDING A DONOR

Your medical team will look for a donor whose HLA type is closely matched with yours. HLA typing tests will be done on blood samples from you, your brothers and sisters, and occasionally your parents, children, or other relatives. The results will determine whether a relative can be a donor. If not, bone marrow registries or cord blood banks can be checked for a suitable match. Searching for a donor through the NMDP or cord blood registries takes time, so this should be done promptly after determining that a related donor match is unavailable.

Once a possible donor is found, this person will have a medical examination to make sure he or she is healthy. He or she will also give full consent for the procedure. The evaluation will be done before you begin chemotherapy. If cord blood is being used for your transplant, it is sent to the transplant facility before you start chemotherapy.

THE DONATION PROCESS

Before the BMT patient is admitted to the hospital, the donor will have a thorough medical evaluation at the transplant clinic. The evaluation takes about half a day. It includes:

What happens at the donor evaluation process?

- A physical exam
- Blood tests
- A urine test
- A chest X-ray
- An electrocardiogram (for adults)

The purpose of the donor evaluation is to learn whether it is safe for the donor to give marrow or blood stem cells, and whether the donor's cells are safe to give to the patient.

During this appointment, a nurse or other staff person will explain the donation procedure in detail. Donors may wish to bring a friend or family member to take notes, as it is a good time to ask questions.

It is important for donors to understand that they are not responsible for the outcome of the transplant. They can't do anything to make their stem cells "better" or guarantee a good outcome for the patient.

Stem Cell Collection Methods

Stem cells from donors are obtained by collecting bone marrow, peripheral blood, or umbilical cord blood. The easiest method is cord blood collection. Normally discarded after a baby's birth, cord blood is especially rich in stem cells. Many parents donate their babies' cord blood to cord blood banks.

How are stem cells collected?

The other two collection methods—bone marrow and peripheral blood—are more complex. The collection method used depends on the patient's disease and other factors. For child donors (under twelve years or one hundred pounds), marrow harvest is usually preferred.

Harvesting Bone Marrow Stem Cells

Bone marrow is full of stem cells available for harvest. Marrow harvest is done in an operating room under general anesthesia or, sometimes, spinal anesthesia, so the donor won't feel anything during the procedure. Small incisions (1/8 inch long) are made on both sides of the lower back. A needle is inserted through these incisions into the pelvic bones, and bone marrow is removed using a syringe to aspirate (suck) it out.

When enough bone marrow has been

Iliac Crest

Marrow Harvest Needle

Bone marrow is often harvested from the iliac crest of the pelvis using a marrow harvest needle. The procedure is done under general anesthesia, so the donor won't feel anything.

removed (typically a quart or quart and a half for an adult, less for a small child), the incisions are bandaged. No stitches are required. Some donors need to stay in the hospital overnight; most go home the same day. This depends on how the person feels after having anesthesia. Sometimes a donor needs blood transfusions during the harvest to replace the blood being collected. Donors most often give one to two units of their own blood two to four weeks prior to harvest (an autologous donation) and then have their blood transfused back to them during the harvest procedure.

What is it like to donate stem cells?

Donors should arrange for someone else to drive them home from the hospital. The bandage on the lower back must stay in place for at least twenty-four hours after the surgery. After that it's okay to remove the bandage and take a shower. Small strips of adhesive may be on the incision sites; they will fall off over the next week.

After the surgery, the area around the hips may be sore for several days. Mild pain relievers such as acetaminophen (Tylenol) or ibuprofen are usually enough to relieve the discomfort. A fever of up to 101°F for twenty-four hours after having anesthesia is common. If fever persists beyond a day and is accompanied by other symptoms, the donor should call a doctor. Symptoms of infection include extreme tenderness, redness, swelling, and drainage. Infections or other complications are very rare.

Donors should take it easy for a day or two after the harvest surgery. It is normal to feel very tired after bone marrow donation. Most donors feel back to normal after one to two weeks.

Collecting Peripheral Blood Stem Cells

Stem cells may be harvested from the bloodstream rather than the bone marrow. Donating stem cells in this way is similar to donating blood.

Before the stem cells are collected, they are first "mobilized," or pushed out of the bone marrow and into the circulating (peripheral) blood. One of two methods will be used to collect the stem cells: growth factor medication or growth factor medication with chemotherapy (used only in autologous transplant, when the BMT patient is also the stem cell donor). The collection process is sometimes called *leukapheresis,* which means "taking away white blood cells."

- **Growth factor mobilization.** To mobilize the stem cells, a medication called a *growth factor* or *colony-stimulating factor* is given. Growth factors are human proteins that are normally produced by our bodies to stimulate blood cell production and growth. They can increase the number of stem cells in the bloodstream.

  How are stem cells taken from blood?

  The growth factor drug is given as an injection under the skin with a very small needle each day for six to seven days. Some donors feel a little pain at the injection site. Side effects are usually mild and may include general aches and bone pain, flulike symptoms, and low-grade fever. The bony aches may increase after each day's injection.

- **Growth factor medication with chemotherapy.** For some patients receiving autologous transplants, growth factor medication is combined with "priming" chemotherapy. The chemotherapy is usually given for two to three days. The growth factors are then given to accelerate white blood cell recovery from chemotherapy and to mobilize stem cells into the blood for collection. Ten to fourteen days after chemotherapy, the white blood cell count recovers and the number of stem cells in the blood is much higher than normal.

The stem cells are collected in an outpatient procedure called *leukapheresis,* or, more generally, *apheresis.* A blood cell separation machine is used to remove some of the stem cells from the bloodstream.

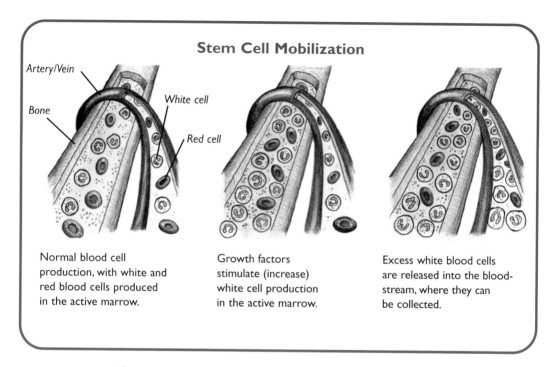

Stem Cell Mobilization

Artery/Vein

Bone

White cell

Red cell

Normal blood cell production, with white and red blood cells produced in the active marrow.

Growth factors stimulate (increase) white cell production in the active marrow.

Excess white blood cells are released into the bloodstream, where they can be collected.

The machine is hooked up to the donor's central venous catheter. The catheter has two separate lumens (tubes) within it. If no central venous catheter is available, two separate IVs may be inserted into large peripheral veins, or a temporary catheter with two lumens may be placed in a neck vein.

What is leukapheresis?

Blood is drawn from one lumen or IV and circulated through the blood cell separation machine. As blood goes through the machine, the white cell portion, which is now enriched with stem cells, is removed for freezing and storage. The blood continues through the machine, and red cells are returned to the donor through the other catheter lumen or IV.

This procedure may temporarily lower the donor's blood calcium level, which may cause a tingling sensation around the mouth or in the hands and feet. To relieve these symptoms, the donor may take antacid tablets that are high in calcium, or calcium may be infused.

The collection process can also lower the donor's platelet count. If this happens, he or she will be watched closely for signs of bleeding.

Each collection will last four to five hours, and several collections may be required depending on the number of cells needed. The hospital will provide snacks during each collection, or donors can bring their own food. Reading, watching television or movies, resting, and talking with visitors can help pass the time.

After the stem cells are collected, the collection bag is sent to a processing laboratory, where the cells are counted and processed. A preservative is added to them and, if the transplant is scheduled at a later date, the cells are frozen.

Some patients are reevaluated after stem cell collection to see how they responded to the priming therapy. This reevaluation (restaging) can include CT scans, X-rays, blood tests, and a bone marrow biopsy.

PREPARING FOR YOUR TRANSPLANT

After stem cells have been obtained (for an autologous transplant) or a donor has been selected and tested (for an allogeneic transplant), you will have chemotherapy and possibly radiation. The purpose of high-dose chemotherapy and radiation is to destroy any remaining cancer and bone marrow cells, so the newly transplanted cells have room to grow. Destroying the bone marrow cells suppresses the immune system, which prevents the patient's body from rejecting the transplanted stem cells. This treatment is sometimes referred to as a *preparative regimen* or *conditioning therapy*.

Why are chemotherapy and radiation given before a BMT?

The preparative regimen most often takes place in the hospital and takes a week to ten days to complete.

Chemotherapy

What are the side effects of chemotherapy?

Chemotherapy will be given by IV through your central venous catheter over several days. The type and amount of chemotherapy depend on the disease being treated, your height and weight, your age, and your general condition. BMT nurses and nurse coordinators will teach you about the specific chemotherapy drugs that will be included in your pre-transplant regimen.

Doses of chemotherapy may be myeloablative or non-myeloablative. When myeloablative chemotherapy is given, doses are high enough to destroy the bone marrow. Non-myeloablative or reduced-intensity chemotherapy requires somewhat lower doses in select cases. While non-myeloablative chemotherapy may be referred to as a "mini-transplant," this is misleading, as recipients are still at risk for significant side effects and post-transplant complications.

The chemotherapy will destroy diseased or cancerous cells, whether they are in the bone marrow or elsewhere. It destroys the normally healthy stem cells in your bone marrow as well. It also suppresses, or reduces the strength of, your immune system and allows new cells to grow.

Chemotherapy will affect normal fast-growing cells, like those in your hair, mouth, stomach, and intestines. Common side effects of chemotherapy include hair loss, nausea, vomiting, diarrhea, loss of appetite, and mouth sores. These side effects are temporary, but some of them may cause mild, moderate, or severe discomfort. For information on the treatment of discomfort or pain, see "Relieving Pain" in chapter 4.

Some of the drugs used in chemotherapy can cause bladder irritation, which may make your urine bloody or cause a burning feeling when you urinate. To prevent this, you'll be given fluids intravenously and you'll be asked to urinate every one to two hours while you're getting this chemotherapy, even through the night.

Some people experience many side effects of chemotherapy, while others have very few. The BMT healthcare team will work with you to keep you as comfortable as possible. Medications can help with nausea and vomiting. You can help yourself by using the stress-reduction techniques that have worked for you in the past. This might mean listening to calming music, expressing your feelings to someone close to you, writing in a journal, or thinking positive thoughts about how the chemotherapy is fighting your disease. Getting out of bed and dressing in your own clothes every day can also help.

It's common to feel tired after chemotherapy. Pay attention to what your body is telling you and get enough rest. When your immune system is suppressed, your energy level is lower and you are more susceptible to infections.

How can I ease the side effects of chemotherapy?

Radiation

Radiation may be given with chemotherapy to destroy diseased or nonfunctioning cells and suppress the immune system. Three types of radiation are used in preparation for a BMT. Depending on the disease being treated, you may receive one of the following:

- **Fractionated total body irradiation (TBI)**—radiation directed at your whole body in a series of doses, where each dose is a "fraction" of the total

- **Total lymphoid irradiation (TLI)**—radiation directed specifically at the lymph system

- **Single-fraction total body irradiation (TBI)**—radiation directed at the whole body in a single dose

Radiation therapy is not painful, but you have to hold very still while it is being given. Each session of irradiation takes five to ten minutes. Children may be given sedation or anesthesia if they are too young to stay still on their own. Family members may go with you to the radiation therapy department, though no one is allowed in the room with you during the radiation treatment.

What are the side effects of radiation?

Short-term side effects of radiation treatment may include nausea and vomiting, diarrhea, hair loss, increased and thickened saliva, low-grade fever, mild jaw pain, and skin rashes. Your healthcare team will help you manage these side effects.

THE TRANSPLANT

The transplant will be given after you have finished chemotherapy and/or radiation therapy. During the transplant, the stem cells that have been collected from the donor (or your own autologous cells) will be given to you. The day of your transplant is called *day zero*. The transplant itself is similar to a blood transfusion.

You may be given medications before the transplant to help prevent side effects such as chills or nausea. Before, during, and after the transplant, your vital signs will be checked to monitor your condition. The stem cells are given through IV tubing connected to your central venous catheter. The transplant usually takes an hour or less.

If the transplant involves frozen cord blood or stem cells, you may feel queasy and have an unusual taste in your mouth during the transplant infusion. Some people also notice an unusual body odor. These reactions are caused by a preservative used to protect the stem cells from damage when they're frozen. The taste and smell will go away in a few days.

After entering your bloodstream, the stem cells are able to find their way to your bone marrow. There they begin to grow and divide. In time, they make new red and white blood cells and platelets. It will be several weeks before the transplanted stem cells produce new blood cells. At this time your body is unable to produce white blood cells, which fight infection. This means you're at greater risk of infection.

What can I expect during the transplant?

Weekly cultures of blood, throat, urine, and stool will be taken to watch for infection. You also will receive medications to prevent infection. If there's any sign of infection, you may have additional cultures taken, and you will be given additional antibiotics. Many people have a fever, which is often the first sign of infection, or chills in the weeks following BMT.

Blood Transfusions

While the new stem cells are growing, you'll need transfusions of red blood cells and platelets to replace those you are not yet producing.

There's always a chance of a reaction to transfusions of blood products. Symptoms include fever, chills, hives, and shortness of breath. If you have had a bad reaction to blood products in the past, tell the medical team. Medications can be given to help prevent reactions.

Will I need a blood transfusion?

Blood products are always tested to prevent certain infections. They are also irradiated to destroy certain cells in the blood transfusion that can compete with the new stem cells and cause transfusion-associated graft-versus-host disease (GVHD).

ENGRAFTMENT

The process in which the stem cells establish themselves in your bone marrow and begin to make new blood cells is called *engraftment*. It usually happens during the first two to four weeks after transplant.

As early as a week after the BMT, your white blood cell counts will be checked. The presence of white blood cells is one of the earliest

How long does it take for new stem cells to establish themselves?

signs of stem cell growth. Particular attention is paid to the neu-trophil count, referred to as *absolute neutrophil count* or *ANC*. Neutrophils fight infection from bacteria and yeast.

A bone marrow biopsy may be done to check for engraftment in the third or fourth week after the transplant. Your white blood cell counts will vary a great deal as the new graft of stem cells establishes itself. Recovery of platelets and red cells is often a bit slower, so you will continue to receive transfusions until you can make enough of these cells on your own.

CHAPTER FOUR

POST-TRANSPLANT COMPLICATIONS

This section addresses possible complications and side effects related to pre-transplant chemotherapy and radiation therapy, as well as other complications that may occur after transplant. Some of these complications can occur after either autologous or allogeneic transplant; others are specific to allogeneic transplant.

In this chapter, you'll read about:

Complications experienced by transplant recipients

> *Mouth sores*
> *Nausea, vomiting, and diarrhea*
> *Anorexia*
> *Bleeding*
> *Fevers*
> *Infections*
> *Liver Complications*
> *Graft failure*

Complications specific to allogeneic transplant

> *Graft-versus-host disease (GVHD)*

COMPLICATIONS EXPERIENCED BY TRANSPLANT RECIPIENTS

Most people who have an allogeneic transplant will stay in the hospital for three to six weeks so the medical team can monitor their progress and watch for signs of complications. Adult autologous transplant patients may be discharged a day or so after the transplant and be monitored in the outpatient BMT clinic.

Almost everyone will have some complications during a BMT. Some of these will be minor and easy to treat, while others may be more challenging or possibly life-threatening. It's important to recognize the signs of complications and promptly report them to your healthcare team so they can be treated quickly.

Mouth Sores

What can I do to prevent mouth sores?

You're likely to develop sores in your mouth or throat after chemotherapy or radiation. The medical term for these sores is *mucositis.* They typically appear three to seven days after chemotherapy or radiation. Some people have just a few sores in their mouths. Others may have sores on their lips and down into their throats. Mouth sores can be very uncomfortable and can affect your ability to eat, drink, or—in the worst cases—breathe or talk. The doctor and nurses will examine your mouth daily. Any pain or tenderness should be reported to your healthcare team.

Several things are done to prevent and treat mouth sores and ease your discomfort:

- You'll rinse your mouth with a salt (saline) solution four times a day while you have low white blood cell counts. Antiseptic mouth rinses may also be recommended to decrease the risk of infection. Avoid mouthwashes containing alcohol.

- You should use tooth sponges instead of a toothbrush to prevent your gums from bleeding.

- You may be given medications to relieve the pain. Narcotics (opioids) such as morphine may be used for moderate to severe pain.

- You should avoid using dental floss for a few months after an autologous BMT. If you've had an allogeneic BMT, you may need to wait longer to floss. Ask your physician when you can floss again.

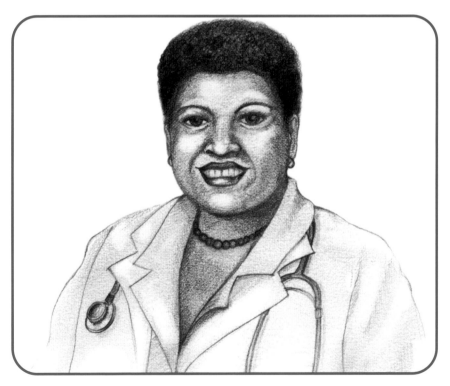

Report complications to your healthcare team so they can be treated quickly.

Relieving Pain

During the transplant process, healthcare team members help to keep patients as comfortable as possible. You may experience some pain or discomfort during the BMT process. One of the more common sources of pain during the transplant is mouth sores, or mucositis. There are a number of things that can be done to either alleviate the pain or make it more tolerable. The methods used to manage pain will depend on how often and how severe the pain is as well as your personal preferences for pain management.

The healthcare team regularly evaluates patient pain or discomfort. Patients can help the team by describing their pain as clearly as possible. One way to help others understand discomfort is to utilize pain scales. Older children and adults may use a type of pain scale that ranges from 0 to 10, with 0 representing no pain and 10 representing the worst pain imaginable. Younger children may be able to identify their discomfort by using a scale with happy faces and sad faces. Infants' and preschool children's discomfort will be assessed using behavioral scales, vital signs, and parental input.

Following are some methods that may be used to increase your comfort. Your healthcare team will work with you to find the method or methods that work best.

Medications

A number of medications can help to increase comfort. For example, narcotics (opioids) such as morphine or other pain-relieving medications are taken by mouth or given through an IV. Some people worry that they will become addicted to morphine or other medications. Treating pain does not cause addiction. Addiction is a psychological dependence on a narcotic and the need to use it for effects other than pain relief. Physical dependence may occur with the use of narcotics, but this is expected; it is addressed by gradually reducing the amount of medication used as discomfort decreases. There are a variety of medications that can be prescribed to increase your comfort. Aspirin is not given for pain, as it can increase your risk of bleeding.

Self-Hypnosis

Self-hypnosis and deliberate relaxation are techniques to help increase comfort during times of pain. By using self-hypnosis or deliberate relaxation, some patients are less likely to be bothered by pain or discomfort. Social workers and other staff members are available to help patients learn these techniques. Relaxation tapes and activities are also available from other hospital staff, such as child family life specialists and chaplains.

Distraction

Distraction—thinking about or doing something else to take your focus off pain or discomfort—may help increase your comfort. Activities that may help include listening to music, talking with family or friends, exercising, engaging in a hobby, or watching movies or television. For pediatric patients, social workers as well as child family life specialists can teach distraction techniques to help the patients prepare for and cope with uncomfortable procedures.

Imagery

Most people regularly use imagery or trances to relax without even realizing they are doing so. You may think of using imagery or trances as "daydreaming." Deliberately using imagery may be a useful way to increase comfort during BMT. Hospital staff can help teach you to effectively use this technique.

Healing Touch

Healing Touch uses purposeful touch to influence a person's energy system. Healing Touch aims to restore physical, mental, emotional, and spiritual balance to facilitate comfort and healing. This technique can complement other medical treatments.

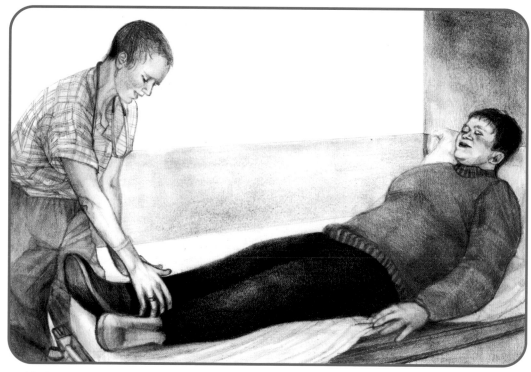

Healing Touch is one of many pain-control methods. Your healthcare team will help you find the methods that work best for you.

Nausea, Vomiting, and Diarrhea

Chemotherapy drugs and/or radiation therapy may cause nausea, vomiting, and sometimes diarrhea. Medications taken after chemotherapy may also make you feel queasy. Tell your healthcare team if an additional medication has made you feel worse or better.

Your healthcare team will prescribe antinausea medications called *antiemetics,* which prevent nausea and vomiting even before you get the first dose of chemotherapy or radiation. Antinausea medications usually are given every four to six hours or as a continuous IV drip. Your medical team may use several different antinausea drugs to control your symptoms.

Nausea, vomiting, and diarrhea can cause problems, including:

- Decreased nutrition. You may need to take intravenous or oral nutritional supplements.

- Weight loss.

- Fluid loss (dehydration).

It can be frustrating as well as physically difficult to live with nausea, vomiting, and diarrhea. It's hard to summon energy and optimism when you're feeling queasy. But remember that these symptoms should improve as you recover. Your healthcare team will help with symptom management during your recovery period.

Anorexia

Chemotherapy and radiation may cause other changes that affect your nutritional status. *Anorexia* is a loss of appetite, which may result from:

- Changes in your sense of taste. Most people describe the taste of food as bland and uninteresting after chemotherapy. Even some of your favorite foods may taste odd to you for a while.

- Nausea and mouth sores. For some patients it takes weeks to regain a normal appetite.

Changes that affect your ability to get enough nutrition will be monitored by the medical team. Your dietitian and pharmacist will regularly check your calorie intake, weight, and protein status to determine what supplements are needed.

For helpful hints on how to cope with nausea, vomiting, diarrhea, and anorexia, refer to the nutrition section beginning on page 68.

How can I manage symptoms like nausea, vomiting, and diarrhea?

45

Bleeding

Until your bone marrow begins making blood cells on its own, you may have problems with bleeding, such as bleeding from mouth sores or nosebleeds. If there are signs of bleeding or your platelet count is low, you will be given a transfusion of platelets. If your hemoglobin count is low (usually below 8.0), you may have a transfusion of red blood cells.

Fevers

Fevers are common during a BMT. A fever may be caused by an infection, a reaction to blood products, or a reaction to medications. Sometimes the cause of a fever is difficult to determine.

How serious is a fever?

Antibiotics are given if the fever is likely to be related to an infection. If the infection is related to the central venous catheter, the catheter may need to be removed or replaced.

When your white blood cell count is very low, your healthcare team will give you intravenous antibiotics at the first sign of a fever over 100.5°F. Antibiotics are started quickly because the immune system is initially not established enough to fight off infection after BMT.

A fever can last from a couple of days to a couple of weeks. Fevers may come and go during your recovery. For most people, acetaminophen (Tylenol) works to reduce a fever and makes them more comfortable. It is extremely important to notify your doctors when you first develop a fever. While acetaminophen can bring the fever down, it also can mask signs that an infection is growing worse. Patients with persistent fevers may have additional tests (X-rays or scans), receive additional medications, or be admitted to the hospital.

Infections

During the first four weeks after your transplant, you are at highest risk for infection, because your white blood cell count is very low. Even organisms that are normally harmless in your body can cause infections after transplant.

Several measures are taken to reduce the risk of infection:

- The air in your hospital room is filtered to lower the risk of airborne infections.

- You will wear a special mask when out of your room or, after you're discharged from the hospital, when coming to the clinic or when in crowds. This will decrease your exposure to infections. Your nurse coordinator or physician will indicate when a mask is recommended and for how long.

- You will be tested for infections frequently during the high-risk period.

- You will be asked to take a bath or shower regularly and to clean your mouth four times a day.

- For some patients, growth factor injections or IV infusions will be used to speed the production of white blood cells.

- Visitors and staff members must wash their hands before entering your room.

- Visitors and staff members may not visit if they have a fever. Visitors must also notify the nurse prior to visiting if they are experiencing other symptoms of infection, such as a cold or rash or diarrhea.

- Visitors will be told not to bring any plants. Molds and fungi commonly found on houseplants and flowers can be dangerous for you as you recover from BMT.

What steps should I take to prevent infection?

47

If you have symptoms of infection, additional tests, cultures, or X-rays may be ordered.

Bacterial Infections

The most common infections after a BMT are from bacteria—primarily organisms that live in your own body. When your white blood cells are suppressed, some of these bacteria can grow and become a problem. Bacterial infections typically develop around your central venous catheter or in your mouth, lungs, or digestive tract.

Signs of bacterial infection include:

- Fever

- Chills, even without fever

- Redness, tenderness, or drainage around the central venous catheter site

- A general achy feeling

Bacterial infections usually respond well to antibiotics. Different antibiotics can be used depending on the type of infection and your history of allergies or reactions to specific medications. Antibiotics are given orally or through your central venous catheter to prevent and treat certain infections.

Fungal/Yeast Infections

Fungi and yeasts normally live all around us without causing problems. But when the immune system is suppressed, a fungus or yeast can grow more than it should. For example, candida, a yeast commonly found in the mouth, intestines, and vagina, can cause sores in the mouth (called *thrush*) as well as more serious widespread infections. Good oral hygiene (mouth care) and antifungal medications can help prevent and treat oral candida infections.

What are the signs of bacterial infection?

What causes fungal infections?

Similarly, aspergillus is a common mold found in many places, often in dust. When it invades the body, it often affects the sinuses or lungs and causes a serious kind of pneumonia.

Fungal infections can be treated with antifungal medications.

Patients with weakened immune systems are especially prone to *Pneumocystis* pneumonia, but specific antibiotic medications are very effective in preventing it. Most patients take this medication twice a day on Monday and Tuesday for about a year after the transplant.

Viral Infections

You may be exposed to viruses while your immune system is suppressed, or a viral infection you had earlier may recur. Viral infections are most common during the first year after a BMT. The most common viruses that affect people after a BMT are cytomegalovirus, herpes simplex, and varicella zoster (shingles).

How common are viral infections?

Cytomegalovirus (CMV) often occurs in people without causing serious disease. You may have had it without knowing it. In a person with a healthy immune system, CMV may cause a fever, flulike symptoms, or no symptoms at all. But after a BMT, when your immune system is suppressed, it can cause more serious illness such as pneumonia or hepatitis.

A blood test will be done before your transplant to see if you have been exposed to CMV. If you or your donor have been exposed to CMV, you will be given antiviral drugs to decrease the risk that CMV could become active after the transplant.

Herpes simplex virus is the virus that causes cold sores and genital herpes. You may have had the virus many years earlier, but it can be dormant for a long time. Herpes can recur with stress, illness, or a suppressed immune system. The mouth sores that are common after transplant will likely be worse if you also have a herpes simplex infection. Genital herpes can also recur during the treatment.

A blood test will be done before your transplant to see whether you have been exposed to herpes simplex. If you have, you will be given antiviral drugs to prevent the infection from coming back.

Shingles is caused by the varicella zoster virus, the same virus that causes chickenpox. Shingles produces painful or itchy sores on the skin, usually on just one side of the body. Early symptoms include burning, itching, and pain in a localized area of the body. Usually within a few days of these symptoms, small blisters will form.

Treating shingles as soon as possible is important to prevent the spread of the infection. Antiviral drugs taken by mouth or intravenously can usually heal the infection quickly. Sometimes the shingles site can be painful (stinging or burning) long after the infection is healed. Prompt treatment can help prevent this long-lasting pain.

Liver Complications

Occasionally, after high doses of chemotherapy or radiation, irritation or inflammation of the liver (called *veno-occlusive disease of the liver*) can occur. Symptoms include:

What is veno-occlusive disease of the liver?

- Jaundice, or yellowish eyes and skin

- Dark urine

- Weight gain/fluid retention

- Tenderness over the liver or on the right side of the abdomen

- Abnormal levels of liver enzymes in the blood

A liver ultrasound may be performed if the medical team suspects veno-occlusive disease of the liver. Most cases get better on their own, but severe cases can be fatal.

Graft Failure

A rare but serious complication of BMT is graft failure. This happens when the new stem cells don't grow or your own immune system rejects the cells. Your old cells may grow back instead.

Graft failure is more common after allogeneic BMT than autologous BMT. Unrelated donor or cord blood grafts may lead to graft failure more often than related donor BMT.

Rarely, after autologous transplantation, the patient's own cells may fail to recover completely. Some patients may need transfusions of red cells or platelets for a few weeks or months.

If no cells grow, it is a life-threatening condition, because your body is not producing any blood cells to fight infection. Sometimes more stem cells can be obtained from the donor. The medical team will talk with you about options.

What is graft failure?

COMPLICATIONS SPECIFIC TO ALLOGENEIC TRANSPLANT

Graft-versus-Host Disease (GVHD)

The immune system is the body's defense against infections. White blood cells circulate through the bloodstream and body tissues, destroying bacteria and other sources of infection. White blood cells called *T lymphocytes,* or *T cells,* are in charge of the immune system. These T cells distinguish cells belonging to your body from those that are foreign and should be attacked. When you have an allogeneic stem cell transplant, the donor cells may recognize your body's cells as foreign and tell the new immune system to attack your normal cells. This is called *graft-versus-host disease,* or *GVHD.*

What is GVHD?

51

The "graft" is the donor's stem cells starting to grow in your body, and the "host" is you. Even if you're a complete match with your donor, you might still develop graft-versus-host disease. GVHD can range from a mild illness to a life-threatening complication. The disease can be acute, developing soon after the transplant, or chronic, lasting for many months after the transplant.

To prevent GVHD, you will be given medications before and after transplant to suppress the immune cells in the graft, which can cause GVHD. These medications, called *immunosuppressive drugs,* are administered at specific intervals. Another method of GVHD prevention is T-cell depletion of the graft, where some T lymphocytes are removed from the stem cell graft before it is transplanted.

Development of GVHD can result in a lower risk of cancer relapse after BMT. The immune attack on normal tissues as a result of GVHD often includes attack on the tumor cells (called *graft-versus-tumor, GVT,* or *graft-versus-leukemia, GVL*).

If GVHD does occur, it can be stressful. Patients are usually expecting to get better just as GVHD emerges. Also, some of the symptoms of GVHD or side effects of its treatment can temporarily affect physical appearance. Some people feel self-conscious when faced with these symptoms.

Many people experience a wide range of feelings when complications such as GVHD occur. Patients may feel sad, worried, anxious, angry, or frightened. Some of these mood and emotional changes can also be caused by the steroid medications used to treat GVHD.

Your healthcare team is available to support you as you cope with the difficult emotions and moods related to GVHD. Sometimes it is helpful to talk to others who have experienced GVHD. At times, antidepressant or antianxiety medications can help.

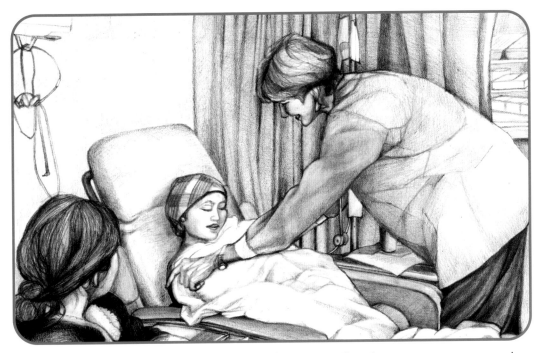

If complications develop after your BMT, your healthcare team will work to treat your symptoms and explain your treatment options.

Understanding the symptoms of both acute and chronic GVHD can help you and your healthcare team detect it earlier. Prevention and early treatment of GVHD are key to a successful allogeneic stem cell transplant.

Acute GVHD

Acute GVHD usually happens during the first three months after the transplant—typically after your donor's white cells start to grow (about three to six weeks). It can affect your skin, liver, and/or gut (gastrointestinal) tissues. GVHD can also increase your risk of serious infection.

On the skin, acute GVHD may appear as a raised red rash over your entire body, but it is often first seen on your face, ears, arms, and trunk. It can cover the palms of your hands or the soles of your feet. It can look like a sunburn and may peel and blister if it is severe.

The transplant team may recommend a skin biopsy to make sure the rash is GVHD and not a reaction to a medication. If a biopsy is done, the skin will be numbed, then a small piece of skin will be removed and examined under the microscope. Once GVHD has been diagnosed, treatment with steroid creams and pills or IV medications will be started.

Liver GVHD causes jaundice (yellowing of the skin and of the white part of the eyes) and abnormal liver function tests. It's usually diagnosed with blood tests, but occasionally a liver biopsy is needed. The healthcare team will check your blood frequently for signs of liver GVHD.

What are the signs of acute GVHD?

Gut GVHD of the intestines causes watery diarrhea. GVHD of the stomach causes nausea, poor appetite, and vomiting. To diagnose gut GVHD, the transplant team will recommend a biopsy of your upper and/or lower digestive tract. This procedure is performed by gastroenterologists, who are specialists in examining the stomach and intestines. Using a flexible, lighted telescope called an *endoscope,* they can examine and biopsy your stomach or intestines. Most adult patients are given light sedation for this procedure. Children usually have heavier sedation or general anesthesia.

Acute GVHD is treated with various medications, including steroids. In addition, the healthcare team will treat your symptoms, which may include diarrhea, nausea, and vomiting. Severe forms of GVHD are treated in the hospital, but some milder forms can be treated on an outpatient basis. Treatment of acute GVHD will take months. Eventually, when the graft accepts your body as home, you may be able to gradually stop taking your GVHD medications.

Chronic GVHD

Chronic GVHD may develop three to six months after a transplant, sometimes even later. It may occur following acute GVHD or it may appear on its own.

Chronic GVHD can affect the eyes, mouth, skin, stomach, or liver. You may develop chronic GVHD while at home recovering from the transplant, so it's important to know the symptoms:

- Dry, scaly, or shiny skin

- Skin rash or discoloration

- Stiff joints or muscles

- Dryness or soreness in your mouth

- Lost appetite, nausea, or weight loss

- Diarrhea

- Difficulty swallowing liquids or solids

- Yellowing of the skin and eyes (jaundice)

- Dry or burning eyes

- Eyes that are sensitive to light

- Shortness of breath or cough

- Vaginal dryness

- Recurrent infections

What are the signs of chronic GVHD?

The skin is the most common area affected by chronic GVHD. At first the skin is red, itchy, and dry. Eventually it becomes discolored, thickened, and tight. Some hair may fall out or turn gray.

Do I need to avoid sunlight?

Sun exposure can bring on chronic GVHD. You should not sun-bathe or use tanning beds after having a transplant. You should wear a sunscreen of at least 30 SPF when you're outdoors.

Keeping your skin moist will help prevent it from becoming overly dry and flaky. Use a gentle, mild soap and a good moisturizing lotion every day. A healthcare provider will prescribe steroid creams to ease itching and burning and to treat GVHD of the skin.

As chronic GVHD can cause stiff joints, people with more severe forms of GVHD may be referred for occupational or physical therapy to help with joint and muscle problems.

Liver abnormalities may also occur in people with chronic GVHD. Yellowing of the eyes (jaundice) and abnormal results of liver tests are usually the only signs. Occasionally a liver biopsy is done to confirm the diagnosis and rule out other possible causes, such as hepatitis or infection.

Chronic GVHD also affects the mucous membranes—the glands in the body that produce moisture, saliva, and tears.

- **Mouth.** Symptoms include pain, dryness, and irritation while eating certain foods. Food might not taste right. Rough spots or ulcers may form in the mouth, on the tongue, and inside the cheeks. Keeping the mouth clean is crucial to decrease the risk of infection. Artificial saliva helps with the dryness.

- **Eyes.** Symptoms include grittiness, burning, and itching. You may not produce tears when you cry. Eyedrops are helpful for reducing dryness and relieving itching. It may help to use these often.

- **Digestive tract (gut).** Symptoms include poor appetite, nausea, difficulty swallowing, vomiting, and weight loss.

- **Vagina.** Symptoms include dryness and painful intercourse.

- **Lungs.** Symptoms include shortness of breath, wheezing, pneumonia, or chronic bronchitis.

Treatment for chronic GVHD uses drugs, such as steroids, to suppress your immune system and decrease T-cell activity. Chronic GVHD usually takes a long time to resolve, with treatment lasting months to years.

Nutritional support, good hydration, physical therapy, and prevention of infection are important for complete recovery from chronic GVHD.

How is chronic GVHD treated?

People with chronic GVHD have a higher risk of infection. If you don't have GVHD, your immune system will be back to its normal infection-fighting strength approximately one to two years after the transplant. With GVHD, your immune system recovery will be delayed until you have completed GVHD treatment and the GVHD is resolved.

While you have chronic GVHD, you will be given antibiotics to prevent certain infections. Contact a member of your healthcare team if you are exposed to chickenpox or shingles. You should not have immunizations with any live virus vaccines until you are off all treatment for chronic GVHD.

CHAPTER FIVE

LIFE AFTER BMT

Your life after a BMT can be good, but it will be different from your life before. Some physical changes require special care, and there may be "late effects" long after the transplant. You'll need to allow yourself a period of adjustment as you recover.

In this chapter you will read about:

Going home

Medications

Clinic visits

Symptoms to watch for

Preventing infection at home

Diet and nutrition

Exercise

Physical changes

Adult sexuality

Relapse

Late effects

Transitioning from patient to survivor

GOING HOME

Your healthcare team will work with you to determine when it is time for you to be discharged from the hospital. Many factors will impact the timing of your discharge, including:

- Side effects or complications that may occur during hospitalization

- Availability of a caregiver to help in the outpatient setting

- Type of transplant

When can I leave the hospital?

In general, people who have an autologous stem cell transplant are discharged from the hospital more quickly than those who receive an allogeneic transplant. Many people who undergo an autologous transplant can leave the hospital the day after receiving their cells. Children and adults undergoing an allogeneic transplant may be in the hospital for four to six weeks following the procedure.

Before you leave the hospital, a number of services will be coordinated. You may need home nursing care, medications, nutritional guidance or support, social services, and physical or occupational therapy. Your healthcare team will explain what you and your caregiver(s) need to know before you leave the hospital. You will learn about medications, for example, and how to properly care for your central venous catheter. Refer to appendix C on page 127 for important questions—and answers—about leaving the transplant center.

After discharge from the hospital, you may experience fatigue and weakness. It is important to have one or more caregivers available to assist you. Caregivers will help you keep track of medications, appointments, and other concerns that may be difficult for you to focus on. Caregivers may also need to provide transportation to and from clinic appointments. If you have housing near the hospital, a shuttle service may be available.

The first few days out of the hospital may be especially difficult. You will have been used to round-the-clock care from experienced medical caregivers. Leaving that behind may make you anxious. Many people find that the transition from hospital to outpatient care is harder than expected, but, with time and support, their comfort and confidence increases.

What should I expect after leaving the hospital?

If your home is far from the hospital, you may be staying near the hospital and away from home for two to three months. Try to make your temporary living situation as "homey" as possible. Stay in touch with loved ones by phone, letters, and e-mail, and take advantage of support groups organized by the hospital.

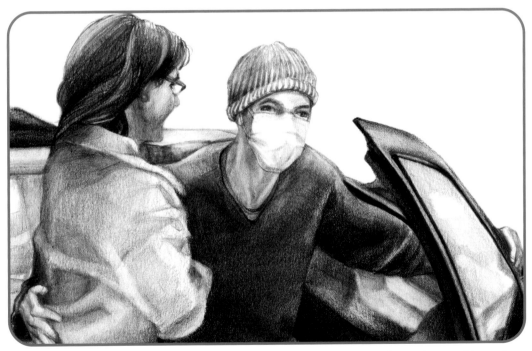

After your discharge from the hospital you will feel tired. You may experience changes in your vision and have difficulty concentrating. Arrange to have a caregiver drive you home.

Remember that you may need a period of adjustment to life after a transplant. You may want to do everything you did before the transplant, but this may not be possible at first. It takes time to recover from a transplant.

How long will it take me to recover?

Recovery is different for everyone. Some people recover soon after a BMT. They go back to work and start participating in their regular activities within a few months. Others recover more slowly, experience setbacks, and may return to the hospital. Some never fully return to their former health and activity level.

Getting back into a normal routine takes time and patience. Consider a part-time schedule when returning to work, school, household chores, and hobbies. It is important to pace yourself and set limits when reconnecting with loved ones, but don't isolate yourself by avoiding friends and family. Improvement occurs gradually as strength and endurance return. Most survivors of BMT say their quality of life is very good overall.

MEDICATIONS

You may need to take a lot of medications when you get out of the hospital. It is very important to take your medications as prescribed. Before you leave the hospital, nurses will give you written instructions and a schedule for taking medications. Medications should not be stopped without checking with your doctor.

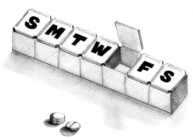

Consider these tips for dealing with medications:

*   Learn the names of your medications, their appearance, and the reason for taking them.

*   Keep a list of known allergies and current medications with you in your wallet or purse.

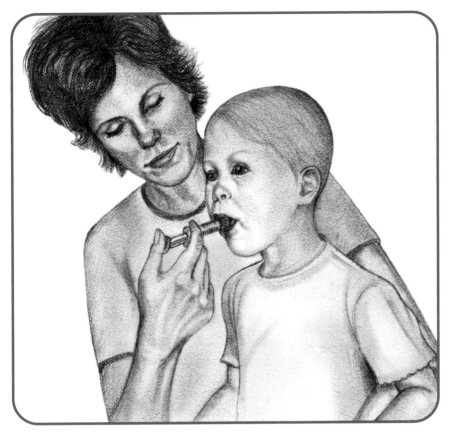

Take medicines as prescribed. Children may require special assistance in taking their medications, such as the use of an oral syringe.

- Get prescriptions refilled five to seven days before running out of a medication.

- Store medications in their original containers in a cool, dry place away from bright light.

- If you have trouble remembering to take your medications, a doctor or nurse can offer ideas on the best way to schedule them. A pill box with different compartments for different times of the day, for example, may help. A medication schedule or chart, such as the one on page 64, is also useful.

Medication Chart

MEDICATION NAME:	Morning	Afternoon	Evening	Night
Dose: Directions:	Comments:			

MEDICATION NAME:	Morning	Afternoon	Evening	Night
Dose: Directions:	Comments:			

MEDICATION NAME:	Morning	Afternoon	Evening	Night
Dose: Directions:	Comments:			

MEDICATION NAME:	Morning	Afternoon	Evening	Night
Dose: Directions:	Comments:			

MEDICATION NAME:	Morning	Afternoon	Evening	Night
Dose: Directions:	Comments:			

MEDICATION NAME:	Morning	Afternoon	Evening	Night
Dose: Directions:	Comments:			

Blood and Marrow Transplantation © 2004 Fairview Health Services

- It is important to tell your healthcare team about any medications you take, including over-the-counter medications, vitamins, and herbal remedies. Do not take herbal remedies without first asking your physician, as some contain substances that can cause infection. Always bring a list of the medications you are taking to your clinic appointments.

CLINIC VISITS

You will go to the clinic for follow-up care often after a transplant. At first you'll go to the BMT clinic every day. The frequency of visits will decrease as your condition improves.

Clinic visits may include blood work, a physical examination, blood transfusions, and IV medications, including antibiotics. If you haven't been able to drink or eat enough, you may be given fluids through an IV.

SYMPTOMS TO WATCH FOR

It's important to be aware of symptoms that might develop between clinic visits. Some symptoms can be very subtle—things you might have ignored before your transplant. After a transplant, however, you should pay attention to anything that doesn't feel quite right. Keep phone numbers for the clinic, the hospital, and your medical team close at hand.

When should I call my medical team?

Call if you experience:

- Fever

- Shaking chills, with or without fever

- Pain or aching

- Cough

- Breathlessness

- A change in bowel habits, or diarrhea

- Loss of appetite

- Nausea and vomiting

- Weight loss

- A new or different rash

- Bleeding that won't stop

- An accident, fall, or other injury

- IV catheter problems, such as redness at the insertion site, difficulty flushing the line, or leaking fluids

PREVENTING INFECTION AT HOME

Just as preventing infection was important during your hospital stay, it continues to be necessary after you go home. Your family members need to understand how to help you prevent infection.

How can I prevent infections?

After your transplant, your immune system will not be able to fight infections normally. For people without GVHD, immune recovery takes one to two years. For patients with GVHD, this recovery can take much longer. Keep this time frame in mind. Even though you may feel well, you still may be susceptible to various infections, some of which might be life threatening.

You and your family can take several steps to help avoid infection during the first one hundred days after BMT or if you have GVHD:

- Wear your mask in crowded areas such as the hospital and clinic. You don't have to wear the mask at other times, but avoid crowds as a general rule.

- Wash your hands frequently.

- Avoid crowds and sick people. Ask friends and family members not to visit when they have a cold or virus.

- Avoid cleaning up animal waste, such as a cat's litter box.

- Avoid people with shingles or chickenpox. If you have been exposed to these, notify your nurse coordinator or BMT physician. These diseases can be serious after a BMT. Pay close attention to changes in your skin color and report any rashes, redness, or blisters immediately to your healthcare team.

- Avoid activities that could lead to a fungal infection, such as repotting plants, chopping wood, yard work, farm work, lake swimming, and visiting construction sites.

- Keep your mouth clean, but avoid flossing for a few months after an autologous BMT; if you've had an allogeneic BMT, you may need to wait longer to floss. Ask your physician when you can begin flossing. Autologous transplant patients may floss once their white blood cell and platelet counts are normal.

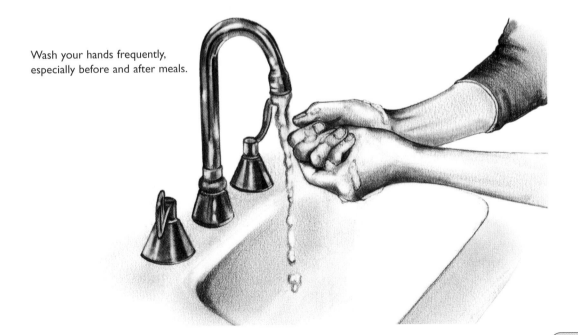

Wash your hands frequently, especially before and after meals.

DIET AND NUTRITION

Nutrition is an important component of your care before, during, and after your BMT. Physicians, nurses, dietitians, and pharmacists are involved in making sure that your nutritional care is optimal while you are a patient. Patients and families need to be involved in this care, too. You can help ensure that your nutrition is adequate in the following ways:

- Make sure that we know your special needs. A dietitian will see you in the hospital (or before hospitalization, if necessary) to assess your nutrition and dietary needs. If you have food intolerances, allergies, or concerns, ask your nurse to inform your dietitian so that we can accommodate you.

- Dietitians will work with you during your recovery to optimize your diet. This may include using special nutritional supplements, adjusting your diet with regular foods, providing snacks between meals, and having foods available at the nursing station for you.

Your eating plan should include the foods you enjoy.

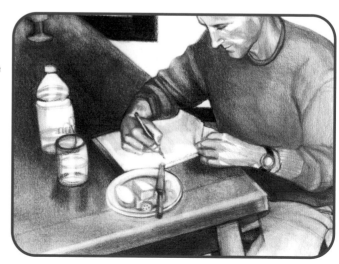

- There may be times when you will not be able to eat enough to maintain yourself. During these times, nutrition may be provided to you directly into your bloodstream (called *total parenteral nutrition,* or *TPN*) or through tube feedings into the stomach or small intestine. Nutrients are needed to avoid infection, repair tissues (like skin, muscle, and blood), and maintain strength.

What happens if I can't get enough nutrients?

- There are many ways to evaluate your nutritional status. Some things we will look at are:

    Intake of nutrients. Amounts consumed or provided by TPN or tube feedings are compared to the estimated amounts needed for maintenance, growth, or replenishment.

    Weight. Your weight may be altered by tissue loss and also by fluid (water) changes in your body.

    Strength. Lack of exercise and lack of nutrients will affect muscle strength. It takes both to regain strength.

    Serum proteins. Serum albumin and transferrin are both used to help assess protein status.

    Other serum levels. Levels of nutrients/electrolytes will be monitored to help assess your status. These include glucose, sodium, potassium, calcium, phosphorus, magnesium, and others.

- Problems can arise, making it difficult to reach an adequate nutritional intake. Sometimes it will not be possible to reach your goals with oral intake, but it is helpful to continue trying. Even while getting intravenous TPN, food intake is still an important part of your recovery process.

- When you are discharged from the hospital, make sure that you are prepared for nutritional support. You may need to continue TPN or tube feeding. If you are able to eat but are not yet able to consume enough nutrients for recovery, you should plan on continuing calorie counts at home. Have some information on the calorie and protein content of foods available, so you know what to try to consume. You will also want to talk to a dietitian before you go home if you have any questions about what you will tolerate or what your nutritional goals are.

What if I have problems eating?

- Remember that your brain and your GI tract are connected. It is not uncommon for your mind to have a great effect on eating problems, even when you are feeling well. You may remember foods that you ate when you were nauseated in the past, and this may make it difficult to try them again. You may be anxious about eating anything because you haven't tolerated food well. You may be sick of people trying to talk you into eating anything and everything. You may feel that food is one of the last things that you can control, and you might resent others for trying to make you eat. Sometimes relaxation or hypnosis may help you return to normal feelings about eating. This may be more effective than medication.

- Talk with your physician or other healthcare professionals about any herbal or dietary supplements that you are thinking about taking. Some herbs and nutrient supplements are not recommended. For other supplements, there may be limits to how much you can use after BMT.

Helpful Hints for Possible Eating Problems

Nausea and vomiting:

- Eat small, frequent meals or snacks instead of large meals. Six small meals may be better tolerated than three large meals. An empty stomach may bring on more nausea.

- Try cold or room-temperature foods, especially if odors are a problem. Cold entrees may be better tolerated than hot ones.

- Try carbonated beverages, such as lemon-lime soda or ginger ale, to help control nausea.

How can I eat if I feel sick to my stomach?

- Mildly flavored, less aromatic foods may be better tolerated: watered-down juices, gelatin desserts, custard, dry cereals, crackers, toast, and potatoes.

- It may help to avoid highly spiced foods or stomach irritants, such as caffeine, pepper, chocolate, and tomato products.

- Liquids may be better tolerated between (not with) meals. Try to separate solid foods from liquids by one hour.

- Avoid cooking odors if they make you nauseated.

- Avoid high-fat, fried, and greasy foods if they bother your stomach. This may include changing from whole milk to skim milk, cutting down on fast foods, and avoiding chips, bacon, sausage, margarine, butter, salad dressing, mayonnaise, ice cream, and pastries.

- Loose clothing may make you feel more comfortable.

- Relaxation techniques may help. If these techniques do not work for you, antinausea medications can be used.

- Exercise and go outside as tolerable. Exercise and getting fresh air may help you feel better.

Sore mouth or throat/swallowing difficulty:

What can I do if
it hurts to eat?

- Try blended, smooth, and creamy foods, such as eggs, soup, casseroles, cheesecake, ice cream, pudding, or smoothies.

- Avoid acidic, spicy, or rough foods as well as hot or cold temperature extremes.

- Use straws to drink liquids and avoid contact with mouth sores. A cup or glass may make it easier to consume soups.

- Tilt your head backward or forward to make swallowing easier.

- After meals, rinse with a mild mouthwash to freshen your mouth (mix 1 teaspoon baking soda, 1 teaspoon salt, and 1 quart water; or combine 1/8 teaspoon baking soda, 1/8 teaspoon salt, and 4 ounces water). Avoid commercial mouthwashes, as they may irritate your sore mouth.

Dry mouth:

- Sip juices or other fluids throughout the day.

- Use butter, gravies, sauces, mayonnaise, and salad dressings to moisten food.

- Dunk or soak dry foods in liquids.

- Suck ice chips, sugar-free candies, or Popsicles, or chew gum.

- Artificial saliva may help keep your mouth moist.

- Use good oral care and rinse your mouth frequently.

Loss of appetite (anorexia):

- Mealtime should be as relaxed as possible. Try taking a walk before meals. Fresh air may help your appetite.

- Make your biggest meal with high-calorie and protein foods when you are the hungriest. Often this will be in the morning, but it could be any time of the day.

- Keep a variety of high-calorie and protein snack foods on hand, such as cheese and crackers, muffins, nuts, granola or granola bars, puddings, and carbohydrate or protein nutritional supplements.

- Make an effort to eat regularly. You may only be able to take a few bites at a time, but it is important to get back to your usual eating schedule.

What if I've lost my appetite?

- Use ready-to-eat, easily prepared food and freeze meals ahead of time whenever possible.

- Add over-the-counter vitamins to your diet, but only with the approval of your dietitian or physician.

Constipation:

- Drink plenty of liquids. Tea, hot lemon water, and fruit juices can be effective.

- Exercise as simple as walking may help with bowel regularity.

- High-fiber foods may be helpful, but only if fluid intake is adequate. High-fiber foods include whole-grain and bran breads and cereals, dried beans and peas, nuts, dried fruits, and fresh fruits and vegetables.

- Make an effort to eat regularly. You may only be able to take a few bites at a time, but it is important to get back to your usual eating schedule.

- Take over-the-counter laxatives only with the approval of your doctors or nurses.

Diarrhea:

Diarrhea may be caused by a variety of factors, including chemotherapy, radiation therapy, infection, antibiotics, GVHD, food intolerance (such as lactose intolerance), and emotional upset. The most useful solution will depend somewhat on the cause of the

73

problem, which the medical team will work to address. While the following suggestions may help control diarrhea, keep in mind that it may not be controllable until the cause is treated, and you may or may not be able to tolerate small amounts of food.

How do I
control diarrhea?

- Eat small amounts of food at one time. Take solids and liquids at separate times. Try to maintain an adequate intake of fluids. Ask your physician, nurse, or dietitian how much fluid you should drink each day. Fluids at room temperature may be better tolerated than hot or cold fluids.

- Avoid greasy or fried foods if they increase your diarrhea.

- Limit foods containing caffeine—coffee, strong tea, cola or other soda, and chocolate.

- Reduce stomach gas by chewing foods slowly and avoiding gum, carbonated drinks, dried beans, onions, foods in the cabbage family, nuts, and highly spiced foods.

- Some foods may be better tolerated than others, including yogurt, rice, cream of wheat, cream of rice, ripe bananas, smooth peanut butter, white bread, cheese, cottage cheese, well-cooked eggs, and baked or broiled chicken, turkey, lean beef, pork, or fish.

- Avoid dairy products if you are lactose intolerant. Lactose is digested by an enzyme called *lactase.* Some people lack this enzyme, which results in diarrhea or gas and cramping. This may be temporary (especially in conjunction with other treatments such as radiation therapy) or permanent. In this situation, small amounts of lactose may be tolerated. Cultured milk products, like yogurt, are usually well tolerated. Lactose-containing foods include milk, foods cooked with milk (cow or goat), cottage or cream cheese, and ice cream. Aged cheeses do not contain lactose. If you are lactose intolerant, you can use a lactase supplement added to foods or taken separately. You can also purchase lactase-treated milk (Lactaid).

Suggested Food Progression

After having problems tolerating foods for a period of time, you may need to start slowly, trying new foods in stages. Here is a plan that may help you reintroduce foods into your diet. If you tolerate one step, move to the next. If you do not tolerate the new step, return to the previous step for a while until you feel ready to try again.

- **Step 1**—Popsicles, Kool-Aid, Gatorade, gelatin, fruit ice, sherbet, broth

- **Step 2**—crackers or toast dipped in soup, baked or mashed potatoes, plain rice or noodles, broth-based soups such as chicken with noodles or chicken with rice, cold or cooked cereal with nondairy creamer or lactose-free milk

- **Step 3**—yogurt, cottage cheese, cheese, cream soups, chunky soups, scrambled eggs, custard, casseroles, milk shakes, and high-calorie/high-protein nutritional supplements

- **Step 4**—tender meats, pizza, tacos, and chili

Are some foods easier to eat than others?

Food Safety: Handling and Preparation

Bacteria in foods may cause infection. This will be especially serious if you are immunosuppressed and therefore less able to fight infection. Here are some suggestions that will help you avoid food-borne infections.

- Do not keep refrigerated, perishable foods too long. Follow the "use by," "keep refrigerated," and "safe handling" information on package labels. Use refrigerated beef steaks, roasts, and deli meats within three to four days. Use poultry, ground meat, and fish within one to two days.

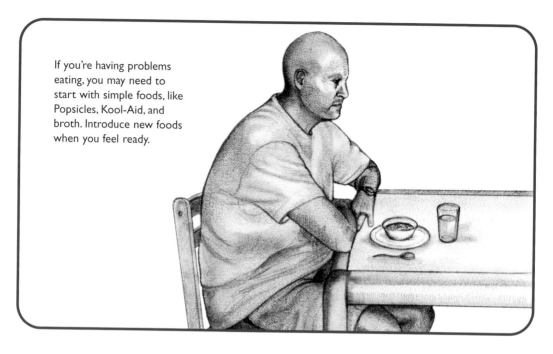

If you're having problems eating, you may need to start with simple foods, like Popsicles, Kool-Aid, and broth. Introduce new foods when you feel ready.

- Make sure that hands, utensils, counters, cutting boards, and other equipment are well washed or sanitized. Wash hands before and after handling food and often when preparing foods, especially between handling raw and cooked foods.

- Wash fruits and vegetables just before preparing for consumption. Storing washed fruits and vegetables in the refrigerator can promote mold growth and cause them to quickly overripen.

- If possible, cut foods to be eaten raw on a clean cutting board reserved for that purpose. Or cut foods intended to be eaten raw on a clean cutting board prior to cutting meats and other foods that will be cooked.

- Keep perishable foods cold until ready to cook or consume. Do not let them sit at room temperature for more than two hours. Do not thaw at room temperature—thaw in a refrigerator or microwave. Refrigerate hard-cooked eggs.

- Roast meat and poultry at an oven temperature of at least 325°F. For beef, lamb, fish, and pork, the internal temperature should reach 160°F. Properly cooked fish should flake easily and be opaque or dull and firm. Poultry should be cooked to an internal temperature of 180°F. Cook eggs until both the whites and yolks are hard. Stuffing should be cooked separately to an internal temperature of 165°F.

- Do not eat raw animal products. Avoid all foods that contain raw or undercooked eggs or egg whites, including cookie dough.

- Serve meat, poultry, and fish on a clean plate. Do not use a plate or other surface that has had raw meat on it. For example, when grilling hamburgers, don't put cooked items on the same plate that was used to carry the raw product out to the grill.

- Once food is cooked, consume it right away, or cool it to 40°F within two hours.

- Consume leftovers in one to two days. Reheat to 165°F, or until steaming or boiling, and stir foods to make sure that they are evenly heated. Items heated in a microwave should also reach at least 165°F. Contrary to popular belief, microwaves do not kill bacteria; higher temperatures do.

- When eating in restaurants or delis, be sure that foods have been handled properly. Hamburgers should be well-cooked; they should not be pink or have pink juice. Salad bars should have a clean, sanitary appearance, with foods either cold or steaming hot. If handling raw meat away from home, make sure to have a method to clean your hands after handling.

Calorie Counts

You may need to keep track of your calorie intake after discharge from the hospital. If so, make sure that you have materials for recording your food intake. Write down all foods and fluids consumed so that your record will be accurate. The dietitian may work with you to identify and monitor your nutritional goals.

Questions

If you have any additional questions, you may call your dietitian after discharge.

EXERCISE

When should I start exercising again?

The idea of exercising may not be very appealing after a BMT, but exercise helps in the recovery from any illness. Easing back into a regular exercise routine helps with physical stamina and flexibility. Often, people who exercise regularly tend to feel better about themselves and their lives than those who do not.

Before starting any exercise program, it is important to talk with your doctor about your limitations. You may be referred to a physical therapist who can help you set up an individualized exercise program.

You may still feel tired and weak from your chemotherapy, radiation, or medications. Nevertheless, it's important to begin exercising—very slowly. Exercise bikes may be available on the unit for use in your room. Or try walking, which is one of the best exercises anyone can do. You can start walking immediately after your BMT, setting your own pace. No special equipment is needed, other than supportive shoes and comfortable clothing. If your physician or the nursing staff permit you to leave your room, you can begin walking while you are still in the hospital.

Once at home, you should continue your walking exercise. Some people find it helpful to choose a specific time of day to walk, then stick to it. Pick a time when you feel the most energy. A morning person, for example, may consider walking right after waking as a healthy start to the day. Those who are not morning persons should walk in the mid-afternoon or evening.

If having a walking partner will help you stay on an exercise program, try to find someone who walks at about the same pace as you. On the other hand, some people enjoy the solitude of walking alone. Listening to music while walking can make the exercise more enjoyable.

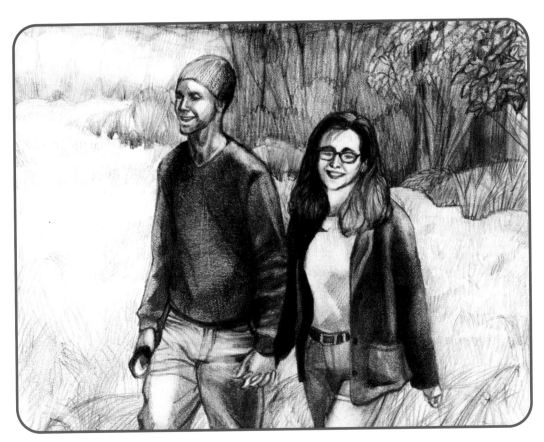

Walking is one of the best exercises anyone can do.

If walking isn't a realistic or comfortable option, a physical or occupational therapist may be able to identify a better type of exercise for you. No matter what activity you choose, it's important not to exercise to the point of feeling pain. Build up slowly, increasing your pace and duration. It's also important to set realistic goals that accurately reflect your energy levels.

PHYSICAL CHANGES

During the months after your transplant, changes may occur in your body and self-image. You may look in the mirror and wonder if your old self will ever return. If hair loss has occurred, it may be growing back slowly. Your face, hands, and feet may look puffy.

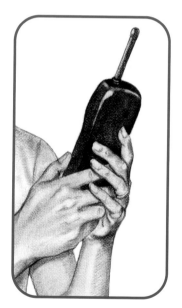

Call your nurse coordinator or attending physician about any physical changes or persistent or worsening symptoms.

Steroid drugs may cause fluid retention and weight gain. The puffiness will disappear as the steroids are reduced. If you are taking steroids for GVHD, you can help control the puffiness by limiting your salt intake. Don't add extra salt to food and don't eat foods that are high in salt. Check the labels of prepared foods for sodium (salt) content and avoid those with high levels. Consider using spices to add extra flavor to your food.

Other physical changes could include weight loss, changes in skin color, muscle cramps, difficulty concentrating, problems sleeping, eye problems, infections, numbness in the feet and hands, and excess hair growth on the legs, face, arms, and trunk. Discuss any physical changes with your medical team.

ADULT SEXUALITY

Sexuality is an expression of one's individuality. The extent to which a transplant affects one's sexual life varies dramatically from person to person.

It is important to check with your transplant doctor to see if there are any restrictions on resuming sexual activity. You may find it difficult to discuss sex with your doctor, but remember that this information may be very important to your overall well-being. Talk to your doctor about any concerns you may have related to sexual issues and recovery.

If you are less interested in sex after your BMT, it could be because you continue to fatigue easily or have a tendency toward nausea, which can suppress interest. Remember that it's okay to go slowly. Sex is not limited to intercourse. You and your partner can share many intimate moments, such as hugging, kissing, holding each other, and gentle touching.

Some people resume an active sex life fairly soon after a transplant. With renewed hope for survival, these patients may feel better about sex than they did before the therapy and transplant.

Others find that their sex life has changed dramatically. Chemotherapy, radiation, and medications may reduce interest in sex. The side effects of treatment may change a person's body, making him or her self-conscious about sex.

One of the best things to do to make sex a safe and vital part of your life is to get into healthy physical condition. Exercise will improve your overall condition and help you feel more confident and positive about your body. This may help to increase your interest in sex, too.

When can I resume sexual activity?

Pay attention to your moods. What causes you to feel blue? What makes you feel good? Are you in a better mood after eating or prior to eating? Do you have a slump just before you go to bed at night? If you're sensitive to your moods, you may be able to take advantage of the times you feel good.

In a relationship, it's important to talk openly about feelings and concerns. Even with the best intentions and honest communication, it may take awhile to get back to a sex life that feels comfortable.

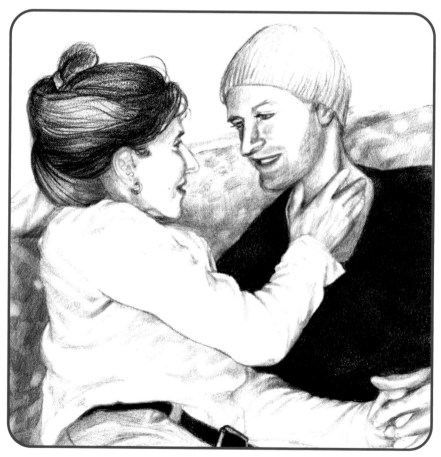

You and your partner can share many intimate gestures—hugging, kissing, holding each other, gentle touching.

Begin slowly and patiently, gradually increasing your activities. Don't try to push sexual activities. Sex may need to be redefined, at least for a while. At the same time, pay attention to whether withdrawing from sex may be due to fear, low self-esteem, or depression.

Women may experience symptoms of early-onset menopause, which can result from chemotherapy and radiation. These symptoms can include hot flashes, vaginal dryness, mood changes, and irritability. Symptoms should be discussed with the physician. Some hormone changes for women and men can be helped by replacement therapy using pills, skin patches, or creams.

For patients who continue to be uninterested in sexual activity, there is help. Physicians may prescribe medication that will help stimulate interest. Professional counseling may be helpful, too.

RELAPSE

Unfortunately, some patients who receive BMT for cancer may experience recurrence of their cancer (relapse). If relapse occurs, it is usually not seen for at least several months post-BMT. You can discuss various treatment options for relapse with your BMT physician. Some patients may be offered a second BMT, while others may receive donor lymphocyte infusions (DLI). New relapse preventative strategies, such as tumor vaccines, are being studied for specific high-risk diseases.

LATE EFFECTS

While some side effects of chemotherapy and radiation may persist, others may not appear until months, or even years, after the transplant. These are referred to as late effects. The list of possible late effects is long, but people usually don't experience many of these problems.

What are the long-term effects of chemotherapy and radiation?

83

Lung Problems

If you have GVHD, you are at risk of developing lung disease, such as recurrent bronchitis, pneumonia, restrictive lung disease, or progressive bronchiolitis obliterans, which can cause shortness of breath or wheezing.

Cataracts

Patients who have undergone BMT are at greater risk of developing cataracts (clouding of the lens of the eye). The increased risk is due to chemotherapy and radiation given before the transplant and the steroids given afterward. People most at risk of developing cataracts are those who have had radiation treatment to the head and eyes, which includes those who have had total body irradiation (TBI). Cataracts can be treated with eye surgery.

Fertility Problems

Chemotherapy and radiation may affect your ability to have children. Young children are less likely than adults to become infertile after a BMT. The kind of chemotherapy received before BMT and the strength of the drugs will also affect one's chances of infertility.

Will chemotherapy and radiation affect my fertility?

Men may want to store their sperm before the transplant. A sperm bank will freeze and store sperm for later use. For women, the issue is more complicated. Not every woman going through BMT will become infertile, but it is a common occurrence.

After a transplant, many women will stop having menstrual periods and begin menopause. Hormone replacement (of estrogen and progesterone) can prevent symptoms such as hot flashes, vaginal dryness, and weak bones (osteoporosis).

Some men may need male hormone (testosterone) replacement to maintain muscle, bone strength, and sex drive. This will not restore sperm production or fertility, however.

Learning that you may lose the ability to have biological children can be devastating, but that concern has to be weighed against the need for therapy that can save your life. It may be helpful to investigate medical options for infertile couples, such as sperm or egg donors. Many people find other ways to become parents or have children in their lives, including adoption, foster parenting, mentoring, and spending time with extended family.

Growth and Development in Children

High-dose chemotherapy and radiation can affect the growth and development of children. How much they are affected depends on the combination of drugs and the amount of radiation used. Steroids used to treat GVHD also slow growth.

Slowing of growth and development is common among children who have not started active puberty at the time of their BMT. After having a BMT, children may take longer to reach sexual maturity. Normally, children start a growth spurt during adolescence, but some children who go through chemotherapy and radiation may not have this spurt, or it may be delayed. Radiation can also affect the growth of bones in the face and teeth.

How might chemotherapy and radiation affect children?

Radiation sometimes causes changes to the brain. Some young children who have a BMT will have learning problems a few years later. The children most likely to be affected are those with leukemia, whose treatment includes radiation to the brain. The older the child is at the time of treatment, the less likely he or she is to have learning problems later.

Children whose development has been affected by chemotherapy and radiation may have problems very similar to those of children with learning disabilities. Many parents find that the same strategies used for children with learning disabilities, such as memory aids, can help children who have had a BMT.

Bone Loss (Osteoporosis)

Chemotherapy, radiation, nutritional deficiencies, steroid therapy, and hormone deficiencies can all cause loss of bone strength. This can increase your risk of bone fractures or large joint problems (affecting the hips, knees, or shoulders). Your healthcare team will monitor your bone strength. Medications and vitamins, including calcium supplements, may be advised.

Secondary Cancers

For a small number of people who have had a BMT, a new, second cancer may develop. Increased risk of cancer is thought to be caused by the chemotherapy drugs and radiation given during the preparation for BMT.

Though secondary cancers are uncommon, the transplant team will monitor your recovery for the development of these cancers.

TRANSITIONING FROM PATIENT TO SURVIVOR

As part of recovery in the months following the transplant, you will make a mental shift from patient to survivor. This shift will add to your quality of life. There are some things patients can do to help make this transition.

- **Believe you will stay alive.** You will enjoy a richer, happier life if you begin your recovery period with this in mind.

- **Set realistic goals for yourself.** Don't aim for goals that are so difficult that you will become discouraged when you can't meet them.

- **Take one day at a time.** Don't look six months into the future—think about what you'd like to accomplish today.

- **Keep a sense of humor.** It will help both you and those around you.

- **Have things other than your disease and transplant treatment in your life.** While your recovery is the most important thing in your immediate future, your life also includes friends, family, hobbies, activities, and perhaps work. Keep abreast of what's happening in the news. Talk to the neighbors. Remind yourself that life is full of interesting things.

- **Take control where you can.** There's much that you can't control, but pay attention to the things you can. They may be as simple as planning your own meals or as complex as developing a new financial plan for your family.

- **Think of yourself as well, not sick.** This may seem difficult, especially when you are first released from the hospital. But you move into a different kind of future when you think of yourself as well rather than ill.

- **Celebrate successes.** It's easy to focus on what's not happening in the way that you wish or as rapidly as you would like. Celebrate each small step of your recovery, and encourage others to celebrate with you.

How can I start thinking of myself as a survivor?

CHAPTER SIX

EMOTIONAL HEALTH

You may face real extremes of emotion when your illness requires a BMT. Your life may be threatened, but the transplant offers hope of survival. This section identifies the potential emotions you may feel, the importance of recognizing emotions, and strategies for maintaining a positive outlook.

In this chapter, you will read about:

Emotions

> *Anger*
> *Fear*
> *Loss of control*
> *Depression*
> *Denial*
> *Isolation*

Coping with mortality

Spirituality

Connection to the donor

Family and friends

You and your caregiver

EMOTIONS

As you go through BMT and recovery, be aware of your mood swings. Ups and downs are common. There may be days when you feel overwhelmed, unable to be "strong." Sometimes your feelings will change with your physical condition. On days when you're feeling better physically, you may feel more optimistic and up. If you're in pain, you may feel depressed or angry.

Are my mood swings normal?

But it's not always that simple. You may find that even when you are feeling good physically, your mood is low. The reverse can also be true—some people find peace and happiness even in the midst of physical pain. Are you "wrong" if you are depressed? Are you "good" if you manage to be optimistic and positive even while in bad shape physically?

Accept that all of your feelings are okay—there are no right or wrong feelings. What's important is to acknowledge them and find ways to express them. Talk to people or find an outlet through creative activities such as writing, music, and art.

Anger

"Why me?" This is a natural reaction for many people who become seriously ill. It's not fair that you developed a life-threatening disease. Children experience anger as well. Parents may have to help their children find ways to cope with this anger.

It's okay to feel anger, but it's not fair to take it out on other people—your spouse or partner, your parents, your doctors. Try directing your anger at your disease: "Okay, cancer, I'm not going to let you get me down. I'm going to beat you." In this way, your anger may be an incentive to help you follow your medical team's instructions and to make it through any complications of your treatment.

Holding on to anger for a long time can make you feel even worse. It's best if you can recognize anger and do what you can to let it go, whether that's talking it out, making a painting, or punching a pillow.

Fear

Your first reaction on learning you need a BMT may be fear. This is completely normal. We tend to be most afraid of the things we don't know. Start out by getting more information. Ask your doctor to explain your condition. Look for books about your disease and discuss what you read with your doctor.

The people who care for you during your treatment are so familiar with your illness and the therapies involved that they may not realize when you don't understand something. Stop them when you don't understand. It's helpful to have a friend or family member with you when you talk to the medical staff to take notes and help you ask questions.

Talk to your spouse, partner, or others who are close to you and let them know what you are afraid of. They can help you get information and keep a good perspective. A support group also may help. It's often comforting to meet people who are worrying about the same things you are—and learning how to overcome those fears.

How can I cope with fear?

You may not be able to completely rid yourself of fear. Fear is a natural response to a serious illness, a long recovery, or even the possibility of death. You may also be afraid of the pain you might feel during your treatment. Address your fear through talking with caregivers and staff. Social workers and chaplaincy services can help you find ways to manage or cope with fear.

Loss of Control

One of the most difficult experiences for some people in your situation is the sense of not being in control. You may be more tired, more dependent on others, or you may have to do things on someone else's schedule. As you recover from your transplant, you will develop a greater sense of control over your life and activities.

You may not be able to do everything for yourself right away, but knowing that your caregivers can help can be comforting. Trusting in your friends, your family, and your healthcare team can help you achieve your care goals.

Depression

Depression can sneak up on you. You think you're doing okay, handling everything pretty well. But you just don't feel like yourself. You have a hard time getting interested in the things you used to enjoy, or you feel more tired than usual. You withdraw from your friends and loved ones.

Many of these symptoms are side effects of chemotherapy, radiation, medications, or GVHD. But they also may be signs of depression.

What are the signs of depression?

It's normal for people to feel some depression soon after discharge from the hospital. Depression is not just in your mind—it's a combination of emotional and physical changes. It isn't something that you can talk yourself out of. If you are depressed, you may need help to handle it.

The first step is to recognize that something is wrong. Talk with your doctor about how you're feeling and what physical symptoms you are experiencing. Your doctor can help determine if your medications or your disease are responsible for the symptoms. If your doctor suspects that you are depressed, he or she can help you figure out the next step. This might mean a referral to a psychologist, psychiatrist, or social worker for counseling and possibly a prescription for an antidepressant medication.

People who are depressed often don't recognize it themselves. If people close to you mention that you seem to be acting differently, don't brush it aside. They may be trying to help you. Talk about how you're feeling and ask what they've observed. If they describe symptoms of depression, talk to your doctor.

What is the treatment for depression?

Symptoms of depression include:

- A sad mood or empty feeling that doesn't go away

- Sleeping too much

- Sleeping too little, or waking frequently and not being able to get back to sleep

- Not enjoying things you used to like

- Eating too much or too little

- Losing or gaining weight

- Feeling irritable or restless

- Feeling tired, or lack of energy

- Feeling guilty, hopeless, or worthless

- Thinking of suicide or death

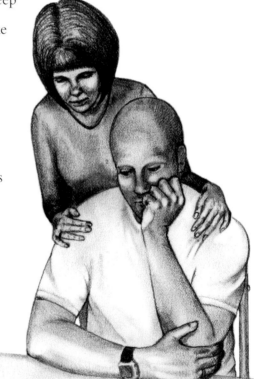

Denial

Some people who learn they have a serious disease will react by not reacting. This is often an attempt to protect themselves from over-whelming information. They ignore their doctor's recommendations and may be careless about taking medications or refilling prescriptions. It's as if they think that if they don't admit they have a serious disease, it can't really hurt them.

Make sure you're not dismissing the seriousness of your situation. It's one thing to keep a positive attitude; it's another to pretend that you're not really ill. Even though it may be difficult or frightening, it's important to address symptoms and problems directly and quickly.

Isolation

All of us need some connection to other people—a spouse or partner, friends, coworkers, family, a therapist. When you're facing a serious medical procedure and the emotions that go along with it, the need to talk to others can be very strong.

How can I talk about my feelings with others?

Good communication doesn't always come naturally. Your need to talk might be overwhelming to someone close to you, or you may feel frustrated that the person you're talking to doesn't seem to be listening. The following ideas include steps you can take to help you communicate well:

- **If you feel like you need to share some of your deepest thoughts, tell your spouse or friend that you need to talk and ask when a good time might be.** If you're telling your concerns to someone who is distracted, both of you are likely to feel frustrated.

- **Let your listener know what you want from him or her.** If you simply need a sympathetic ear, tell the person you need to vent but that you would rather not receive any feedback at the moment. If you are looking for advice, ask for it. If you want to talk about something other than your transplant, just say so.

- **Be honest with others and yourself.** It is important that you tell others how you are feeling—even if it may worry them. Not being honest with others builds a wall between them and you.

- **Practice listening as well as talking.** Remember that people close to you have their own worries and concerns. Maybe your spouse or partner would like to tell you about his or her fears about your disease. Let others know you're still there for them.

- **Listen to yourself.** It's okay to talk to yourself about your disease and your emotions. In fact, talking to yourself is one way to cope with emotions. Give yourself a little "you can do it" speech, but also pay attention to the things you seem to be fretting over. Maybe you can problem solve, finding ways to deal with them by yourself or with the help of others.

COPING WITH MORTALITY

Although much of this chapter and the advice you will get focus on keeping a positive mental attitude and seeing yourself as recovering, some patients will have to face the possibility that things are not going well and that they may die soon. You may have confronted this idea already, but each round of chemotherapy and radiation brought new hope of stopping your disease. BMT offers another hope for a cure. But for some people, the BMT will not be enough.

What if I don't recover from the BMT?

There may come a time during your BMT treatment when further medical intervention seems unlikely to lead to a cure or a return to a meaningful life. When recovery no longer seems possible, you and your family may face difficult choices. The healthcare team, while concerned with the physical aspects of your care, will also help to address your spiritual, emotional, and intellectual needs at that time.

If recovery seems unlikely and you have questions or concerns, the healthcare team is available to talk with you. You may also want to speak with your family, friends, support network, spiritual advisor, social worker, or others. If at any time you wish to talk to the healthcare team about your prognosis or plan of care, you may request a care conference.

Your spiritual or religious background, your family situation, your age, and your outlook on life may all influence your thoughts and feelings about death and your way of coping with it.

If it is clear that you're not going to survive, it may help to find ways to fully appreciate the time you have left. Some people do this by thinking of very practical things. They give away some of their possessions, plan their funerals, and write letters to the people who are close to them. Others deepen their spirituality, perhaps with the help of a clergyperson, friend, or family member. It is important for you to know that there is no one way to cope with the possibility of death. Members of the medical team are available to support and assist you during times of change and uncertainty.

SPIRITUALITY

Many people find that coping with a BMT is more meaningful if they connect with their higher power in accordance with their beliefs. Looking deeply into yourself can help put your life and concerns into a broader perspective.

You may find that reading, studying, meditating, or praying are important to you now. This may be a good time to explore your spirituality. Reading sacred texts or inspirational literature may help you find meaning in a difficult experience.

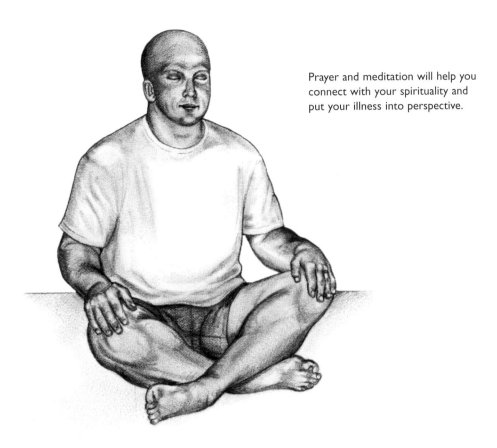

Prayer and meditation will help you connect with your spirituality and put your illness into perspective.

You may feel angry that you have a life-threatening disease. What did you do to deserve this? Haven't you been good enough? These questions and others are normal reactions. Talk with your minister, priest, rabbi, or spiritual adviser about your feelings. Hospital chaplains are also available to offer spiritual and emotional support for you and your family.

CONNECTION TO THE DONOR

If you have had an allogeneic stem cell transplant, you may feel a special link with your donor. This can be a wonderful connection, particularly if your donor is a family member. Indeed, the donor may have given you a second chance at life, and you may feel honored and deeply loved by that gift.

How can I thank my stem cell donor?

And yet, this emotional connection can be complicated. Some people feel uncomfortable owing anything to others. Owing a chance at life is a large debt, and you may feel resentful or guilty at the same time you're feeling grateful.

With an unknown donor, you may wish to find a way to thank this person. You can write letters to the donor even before learning the person's name. During the first year after the transplant, you will not be able to learn the donor's name and you are required to leave your letters unsigned. The nurse coordinator who handles the donor searches will forward your letter at the appropriate time. It is important that the confidentiality of both you and your donor are protected.

FAMILY AND FRIENDS

Families and friends can be especially important to you during your illness, transplant, and recovery. You may feel closer to them than ever before. Your illness may encourage all involved to be more aware of how important these relationships are. On occasion, however, some family and friends will seem to disappear from your life. Usually, this is related to their not knowing what to say or do. Some will return once they work through their feelings.

One frequent cause of stress between patients and their friends and families relates to differing emotional stages. You may be feeling positive and optimistic about your recovery, while your family is concerned that you may die. You may be fearful at a time when they are upbeat and positive. You may feel that your family is too negative or not supportive enough. Your family may want to talk to you about your plans for the future when you are just trying to get through the day. To navigate these situations, you may find it helpful to talk to a counselor, your social worker, or a member of the medical team.

Families face other stressors as well, and you may not have the energy to deal with these while you're recovering. Long hospital stays can cause financial stress. If you are far from home, family members may be separated from each other. Your children may have to leave their regular schools or perhaps live with someone else for a time. For these kinds of stressors there are no quick and easy answers, but many helpful resources are available at the hospital and in your community.

YOU AND YOUR CAREGIVER

The caregiver role is rewarding and stressful. Like you, caregivers feel removed from their normal lives and routines. Caregivers may feel isolated when living away from home, family, and friends. Even if you live near the transplant center, the caregiving role involves taking time from work and other activities. Caregivers may feel burdened or guilty if you are not feeling well and they can't do anything to make you get better. And sometimes it's just difficult to spend so much time together in an unfamiliar setting.

How can I make this easier for my caregiver?

Both you and your caregiver should think about the caregiver's needs. There are several things you can do to make the role a little easier:

- Make sure the caregiver has time off. Other friends or family members can take over the caregiving role for a period of time.

- If possible, rotate caregivers so that one person doesn't have to be there for your whole transplant stay.

- Encourage someone else to take the caregiver out to lunch or out for other activities.

- Plan for the caregiver to get exercise or take walks.

- Encourage your caregiver to attend a support group.

It is normal to have some difficult days with your caregiver. If you have ongoing problems, consider asking for help from the hospital social worker, nurses, or physicians.

There will be good days. This can be a time of new and renewed closeness. Remember that you care about each other and are working together toward an important goal—getting well.

FOR CAREGIVERS

This chapter discusses the role of the caregiver and offers suggestions for taking care of oneself as well as the patient.

You'll read about:

Being a caregiver

Emotional well-being and common feelings
   Fear
   Resentment
   Abandonment
   Sadness
   Depression

Healthy ways to deal with feelings

BEING A CAREGIVER

A caregiver plays a crucial role in helping a patient through BMT and recovery. A caregiver is a family member, parent, or friend who can be with the person receiving a transplant during his or her stay near the transplant center. As difficult as it sometimes seems, finding someone to fill this role is a key component of a full and safe recovery. It is important to start deciding who can fill this role prior to the workup evaluation.

Being a caregiver for someone who's having a BMT can be a life-changing event. If you have offered to be a caregiver, you will be helping someone you care about, a kind of help and giving that may lead to personal growth and added closeness to your loved one. You will need to learn to perform various physical tasks. You also will need to take care of yourself emotionally and physically while trying to support a loved one whose emotions can fluctuate a great deal after this major procedure.

Prepare yourself in advance for the caregiver role. If your spouse, partner, or child is the patient, for example, it is natural for you to become the caregiver, and it is probably something you want to do. But you should be honest with yourself about your strengths and weaknesses and look for help when you need it. You will be called on to provide emotional support, practical tasks, and simple medical procedures for the patient. Get help with these things in whatever way best supports your efforts.

Caregiving requires a significant time commitment. The patient needs help at many different times, for everything from driving to appointments to preparing meals. As the patient recovers the time commitment should ease, but for many weeks the caregiver may need to devote most of the day to the patient's needs. A caregiver's tasks include:

- Providing emotional support and encouragement

- Going with the patient to appointments

- Communicating with transplant team members and gathering information

- Assisting with the scheduled oral and intravenous medications after hospital discharge

- Keeping track of the medications taken after hospital discharge

- Keeping an eye on the patient's condition and identifying any changes or new symptoms

- Caring for the central venous catheter

- Knowing what to do in an emergency

- Calling for medical help when needed

- Communicating with other family members and friends

- Keeping a clean and comfortable home environment

- Helping to prepare or provide meals for the patient

- Providing transportation to and from the treatment center or clinic

- Helping with medical and hospital bills, insurance paperwork, and financial planning for the family

What are the caregiver's responsibilities?

Being a caregiver can shift your role as a family member or friend. Caregivers become extremely knowledgeable and attentive to the tasks that they perform for their loved ones. They are often separated from their own spouses or children during the transplant. Preparing for this will be helpful to the whole family.

If the patient is your spouse or partner, you're probably used to sharing responsibilities and activities and supporting each other. During treatment, however, you may not be able to turn to your spouse or partner for support. He or she will be focused on recovering from the BMT and simply may not have much to give emotionally. Your relationship won't be like this forever, but it may have to be like this for a while.

Being a caregiver for your child is equally demanding. It can shift your primary role from that of parent to that of medical caregiver.

Caregiving is a demanding job, one that can't be done well if you're stressed and tired. There are things you can do to take care of yourself.

How can caregivers take care of themselves?

- The more you know, the more comfortable you're likely to be with the role. Take advantage of the classes and training offered by the transplant program.

- Make sure you take some time for yourself. Get away from the hospital or house once in awhile. Talk with friends. Go to a movie or take a long walk.

- Turn to other people for help when appropriate. Even if you are the main caregiver, other friends and relatives may be able to help with such things as preparing meals or providing transportation.

- Communicate openly and honestly with the patient about your needs as well as his or her needs.

- Take advantage of available resources, such as transplant program support groups, your social worker, or a chaplain or other spiritual adviser.

EMOTIONAL WELL-BEING AND COMMON FEELINGS

When a loved one has a serious disease, the focus naturally shifts to him or her. The patient needs a lot of emotional and physical support through the long treatment and recovery process. It's easy for you—the spouse, partner, sibling, parent, child, or intimate friend—to fade into the background. Friends and other relatives call or visit the person who is ill. All of your conversations may end up being about the patient's treatment and progress.

Sometimes you, too, need a chance to have a good laugh or cry. You need to be able to talk about what's scaring you or making you angry. Sometimes you just need a break.

It's important for you to recognize and talk about your own feelings, but you need to turn to other people besides your loved one. He or she has a lot to cope with and probably can't be as supportive as usual. If your loved one is the person you usually talk to about most things, make an extra effort to find sympathetic, supportive, and helpful listeners.

Some of the emotions you may feel are discussed below. Maybe you'll feel all of these—or none of them. Remember that everyone reacts differently during times of stress.

Fear

You might be fearful about whether your loved one is going to live. You may fear that you don't have the strength or courage to go through illness, treatment, and recovery. Maybe you're afraid you'll be left alone without enough money to keep your home or take care of your children.

You may simply fear the unknown. What happens next? Will you be taking care of an invalid, dealing with death, or getting both of your lives back on track? When will life return to the way it was? Some people are great at handling the most awful circumstances but are uncomfortable in situations where they can't predict the outcome.

The saying that "we have nothing to fear but fear itself" probably seems a bit simplistic for the complicated situation you find yourself in. But fear is crippling. It tends to stop you from doing things that can improve your situation.

Getting information is one of the best ways to deal with fear. It won't take away all your fear, but it will help you control it. If you're worried about money, now is a good time to get the details about your savings and expenses and to talk with a financial adviser or social worker. If you're worried about the treatment, ask the doctor questions and do your own research. Reassurance from others may help.

Tell your loved one something about your fears, but be cautious about sharing too much. Most caregivers have a lot of fears. Knowing that you are not alone with your feelings may be important to you—and may actually help—but your loved one may not be in a good position to support you. Find a support group where you can talk about your fears and hear how others have faced theirs.

Resentment

Is it wrong to feel resentment?

You may have some feelings of resentment toward your loved one, and yet wonder how anyone could resent someone who is ill. You may not want to talk about this feeling of resentment, fearing that people will think it is selfish, insensitive, or mean to resent a loved one who is ill and may die.

But resentment in this situation is not uncommon. Perhaps you blame your loved one for allowing the illness to develop, even when you know that's not what happened. You may resent the time and energy you are expected to give. You might even resent the attention that the patient gets, while you are exhausted. Your life has had many difficult changes since finding out about the disease. You may resent your loved one for these unwelcome changes. It may be that you are resenting fate, your higher power, or the healthy people you know. You may want to shout about how unfair it all is. Why is your loved one ill and not someone else?

You may be experiencing these feelings and have a difficult time expressing them to others. Remember that resentment is a hard emotion to conceal or bury. If you feel it, at some point you are likely to express it—directly or indirectly. If you've bottled up this feeling for a while, it can come pouring out in an ugly way that may be hurtful to others. A better way to cope with your feelings of resentment (or any difficult feeling) is to talk with a trusted friend, a counselor, or others who have been through a similar experience. Your hospital and clinic have support groups and can refer you to counselors or therapists who can help you.

Abandonment

Although you may be spending all of your time—or what seems like all of your time—with your loved one, you can still feel as if you've been abandoned. You can't really be part of his or her life in the same way as before the illness. The patient is on a "journey" of illness. You can't really be part of it if you aren't ill yourself. The patient's full attention is focused on the disease, the treatment, and what this means for the rest of his or her life. Although the person loves you, he or she is "gone" for much of the time—just when you really need support, love, and understanding.

Although your loved one may need a lot of your time, you can take a few hours here and there to be with other friends or family members. Surround yourself with people who care about you. Take breaks from caregiving and ask others to occasionally relieve you. You might, for example, go to lunch with a friend, read a book or newspaper, watch a video, spend time with family, or simply take a walk.

Try not to abandon your loved one emotionally because you feel abandoned. Strive to be close. Do this in positive ways (finding things to laugh about together or reading out loud together, for example). Talk about the evening news or how proud you are of the children. Hold hands and hug and use loving words. Your life together is more than this disease and recovery.

Sadness

What is the difference between sadness and depression?

It is very natural to feel sad when someone close to you is ill. You see one of the most important people in your world going through a rough time. You may be facing the possible loss of this person. There are new emotional and physical demands on you, and it may feel like you are alone.

Things are not normal, and you probably miss normal. You want to pull the blankets over your head and go to sleep. You want to cry. If you need to cry, go ahead and cry. Crying is a healthy release that can make you feel better. If you want to sleep, sleep late when you can. Spend time with friends and family who will understand, comfort you, and be with you in your sadness.

Do try to include some things in your life that make you happy. Go to funny movies (laughter, too, can make you feel better), take walks in pretty places, spend time with friends who are interesting and lively, or read bedtime stories to your children or to someone else's children.

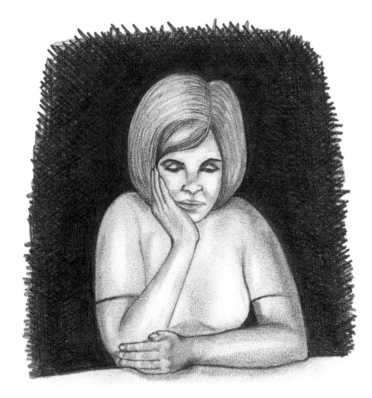

Depression

Sadness and depression are normal, but depression goes beyond sadness. When you are depressed, you tend to feel a sense of hopelessness. You're convinced that things will never be good again.

Some signs and symptoms of depression include:

- A change in sleep habits. You sleep all the time, you wake up too early, or you can't fall asleep.

- A change in eating patterns. You find yourself eating too much, or you don't feel like eating at all.

- Weight loss or gain.

- Lack of energy.

- Loss of interest in things you used to enjoy.

- Feelings of worthlessness or hopelessness.

- Thoughts about suicide.

If you think you may have depression, you need to get help. Depression is a real illness and can have serious effects.

How is depression treated?

People who are depressed don't always recognize that they are depressed. If friends say you don't seem to be yourself or ask if you are depressed, pay attention. They are giving you very important feedback. It may help for you to see a professional to determine whether you are experiencing depression. Counseling, along with medication, could be helpful in treating your depression.

HEALTHY WAYS TO DEAL WITH FEELINGS

It's important to express your feelings, but you don't want to let them get the best of you. Consider some of the following healthy ways to express feelings.

- **Learn or practice deep breathing exercises.** Sit quietly for a few minutes each day and pay attention to your own breathing. Try to clear your mind of thoughts and feelings for this time. Just close your eyes, notice your breath, and be aware of yourself in this moment. This is a beginning form of meditation that may bring you some peace and help you get through each day more easily. If you find this helpful, you may want to learn more about meditation.

- **Talk to yourself about how you feel**—and recognize that it's okay to have these feelings.

- **Talk to other people.** They can give you a reality check and provide support when you need it.

- **Use what has helped you feel better in the past.** If exercise is your way to let out anger, then get to the gym, go for a bike ride, or go for a walk. If pampering yourself helps you deal with sadness, then bring out the bubble bath and the scented candles, or listen to soothing music.

- **Look to your spirituality.** People who have a regular place of worship can find support in going to services. If you are away from home, you may want to find a local place of worship. If your spirituality is more personal and individual, find ways to explore it on your own.

- **Read inspirational books.** A book of meditations or prayer or books about others who have struggled with a loved one's illness can affirm that you are not alone.

How can caregivers cope with their many feelings?

APPENDIX A

ADULT PREPARATION CHECKLIST: GETTING READY FOR TRANSPLANT

This checklist is a guide to help you prepare for your BMT. Some items will not pertain to your circumstances. You may use this list to help you formulate questions for your BMT nurse coordinator, social worker, or financial worker. To contact the organizations listed in this checklist, refer to the Resources section on page 147.

General Advice

❏ Identify someone to assist you during and after your inpatient stay. This person could be a family member or friend. He or she is commonly designated as "caregiver" because he or she participates in your follow-up care. It is necessary to have a caregiver to stay with you after discharge.

❏ To assist your caregiver in understanding his or her role, ask your social worker what is expected. When does the caregiver need to be with you? What types of activities will he or she be asked to perform?

❏ Identify strategies for understanding information about your upcoming treatment. You may want clarification in writing, or you may want to have your caregiver, family member, or friend present to hear information with you. A tape recorder will allow you to play back important information at a later time.

Family

❑ Set up family meetings to talk openly about the transplant and plans you and your family need to make.

❑ If you have children or grandchildren, explain to them in words that they can understand why you are going to the transplant center. You may use books, photos, or videos to help them understand. Your social worker can provide supportive materials.

❑ Talk to your children about what will happen to them while you are in the hospital and recuperating from the transplant. Identify who will be with them, how their schedules will be maintained, and how you will communicate with them. If you want assistance talking with your child or children, contact your social worker or child family life specialist.

❑ Discuss your needs and concerns with your spouse, partner, or significant other.

❑ Consider setting up an appointment with a counselor to assist you and your family in preparing for transplant.

Support Groups

❑ Children may benefit from connecting with others in their age group who have a family member being treated for cancer. Both the American Cancer Society and the Leukemia and Lymphoma Society offer children's groups in many locations. Kids Konnected offers a Web site and a toll-free phone line with simple instructions to help you talk with children about cancer. Your social worker may refer you to other groups at the hospital or in your community.

❑ Support groups for adults and family members often help during stressful times. They provide answers to commonly asked questions, as well as support from others who have been in similar circumstances. To find a support group in the area where you will be staying, contact your transplant center, a social worker, or the local American Cancer Society.

Caregiver

❑ Your caregiver may need to complete routine dental and medical appointments that will come up in the next several months. He or she should refill necessary prescriptions and arrange a method for filling prescriptions while away from home.

❑ Caregivers who are under a physician's or therapist's care should determine how to follow their own care plans while away from home. Have them arrange possible follow-up care near the transplant center. They should also ask healthcare providers what to do if they need professional care while they are away from home.

Before Leaving Home

❑ Prepare a packing list. Think of clothes for different temperatures and seasons, if appropriate. Include some family photos or posters that might brighten your hospital room or temporary living space.

❑ Bring phone lists, addresses, and e-mail addresses.

❑ Arrange how your home or apartment will be looked after while you are away.

❑ Consider how bills will be paid in your absence. When possible, pay bills in advance. Consider checking with lenders about temporary deferments of loan payments due to medical disability.

❑ Have your mail forwarded or arrange to have someone review your mail for you while you are away.

❑ Arrange for someone to care for your pets during your intensive treatment. Most temporary lodging facilities do not have accommodations for pets.

❑ If you have a pet bird or reptile, there may be restrictions on handling your pet following transplant. Ask your physician for guidelines.

Employment

❏ Contact your employer to make arrangements regarding your absence from work. Ask your employee human resources representative to help you understand your rights regarding insurance coverage, COBRA insurance benefits, work disability, and family medical leave.

❏ Ask your physician about the estimated duration of your disability. You may qualify for Social Security Disability Insurance (SSDI) or Supplemental Security Income (SSI). Your social worker or your human resources representative at work can help you understand how these programs may apply to your situation.

Accommodations

❏ Check with your insurance provider to see if benefits cover travel, meals, and lodging for yourself and a caregiver.

❏ Ask your social worker about lodging resources near the transplant center. The National Association of Hospital Hospitality Houses may also offer options. Or call the University of Minnesota Medical Center, Fairview, accommodations office.

❏ Make travel arrangements. You may want to ask a family member if he or she has frequent flier miles available to assist you. Or contact the National Patient Transport HELPLINE Program for resource information. The BMT social workers may be able to provide additional resources, such as airlines that offer discounted fares.

Legal

❏ You may be interested in estate planning, establishing a trust, planning guardianship contingencies if you are a single parent, completing advance directives, or designating powers of attorney. Depending on how complicated your financial or legal affairs are, you may want to consult an attorney who is knowledgeable of financial/family law. Many employers have employee assistance programs that include access to legal advice. You can also contact your local bar association for referral to someone practicing in this area of law.

❑ If you do not share a joint checking account, you may want to designate someone to temporarily handle your financial affairs.

❑ You may want to know your rights under the Americans with Disabilities Act, which protects you against discrimination upon your return to work.

❑ If your minor children will be separated from both parents, you need to give permission for another adult to access medical care for them (emergency or routine) in your absence. Generally, a signed statement will suffice, but you should verify this with an attorney and your child's pediatrician.

Financial

❑ Some organizations offer limited financial assistance to help with costs not covered by insurance. These include The Leukemia and Lymphoma Society, for patients with leukemia, lymphoma, myelodysplastic syndrome, or multiple myeloma, and the Lymphoma Research Foundation, for patients with Hodgkin's disease and non–Hodgkin's lymphoma. Check with your transplant center for additional resources.

❑ The federal government has two income insurance programs available for adults: Social Security Disability Insurance (SSDI) and Supplemental Security Income (SSI). Eligibility is based on a determination by your physician that your disability will last one year or longer. You may qualify to start receiving benefits at an earlier date. Contact your local social security office to apply. If you are covered under your employer's disability plan (short- or long-term), your employer will assist you in determining when to apply. Those who qualify for SSI (based on minimum income requirements) may be eligible for medical assistance that can help cover medical care expenses.

❑ If you are a veteran, contact your VA office to inquire if you are eligible for any programs based on your service record and disability.

❑ Fundraising may be done locally on your behalf. You may want the assistance/expertise of a fundraising organization if you anticipate uncovered medical expenses. For a list of organizations, call the National Foundation for Transplants or the National Marrow Donor Program's Office of Patient Advocacy.

Finding Support

❑ Talk honestly with friends, family members, and colleagues to help them understand the types of support that will assist you and your family during this difficult time.

❑ Support comes from many sources. Reach out to colleagues, neighbors, community organizations, religious or spiritual groups, extended family, and supportive friends.

❑ Go online to find information and connection with transplant survivors. For example, the Blood and Marrow Transplant Information Network provides a number of support services.

Faith/Spirituality

❑ Identify your personal source of spirituality, such as your faith community, meditation, reading, music, walking, nature, or rituals.

❑ If you belong to a faith community, arrange to keep in touch with other members. Members may want your mailing address and e-mail address to send you cards, letters, and messages of encouragement.

❑ You may find connections to your faith community near your transplant center. The chaplains at the center can assist you.

❑ A chaplain is available to you during your time in the hospital.

Adapted from "Preparation Checklist for Adult Patients: Getting Ready for Your Stem Cell Transplant," developed by Caroline Gale, LICSW; Doris Knettel, LICSW; Stacy Stickney Ferguson, LICSW; Janet Ziegler, LICSW; University of Minnesota Medical Center, Fairview, BMT Social Workers; and Kate Montgomery, LICSW, at the Office of Patient Advocacy at the National Marrow Donor Program.

APPENDIX B

PEDIATRIC PREPARATION CHECKLIST: GETTING READY FOR TRANSPLANT

This checklist is a guide to help you prepare for your child's BMT and your stay at or near the transplant center. Some of the suggestions may not apply to your circumstances, and others will help you think about preparations not listed. Please contact your BMT nurse coordinator, social worker, chaplain, child family life specialist, or patient financial representative if you have questions or need assistance. To contact the organizations listed in this checklist, refer to the Resources section on page 147.

Patient

❑ Talk honestly with your child about the trip to the transplant center and explain, in words that your child will understand, why you are making the trip. You may use books or other visuals to help tell the story.

❑ Talk with your child about the plan. You may include details of how you will travel, who will come along, and what will happen with siblings and pets who will be staying at home.

❑ Talk with your child about what will happen when you arrive at the transplant center. Use words and concepts that children can understand. You might include information about where you will be living, where he or she will receive medical care, and what your schedule will be like.

❏ Reassure your child that Mom, Dad, or another identifiable care-giver will be with and take care of him or her for the entire stay.

❏ If you want help talking with your child, ask a social worker or child family life specialist at your local hospital.

❏ Help your child to make a list of things he or she would like to take along on the trip.

Parents

❏ Make necessary arrangements with your employer. Utilize paid or unpaid leave of absence. Speak with your supervisor and human resources department about the Family Medical Leave Act.

❏ You might explore the possibility of maintaining some level of paid work via telephone, facsimile, and computer.

❏ Arrange how your home or apartment will be looked after while you are away.

❏ Consider how bills will be paid in your absence.

❏ Consider having your mail forwarded to your address near the transplant center, or have your mail evaluated and held at home.

❏ Discuss with your spouse, partner, or significant other your own needs and concerns.

❏ Begin to think about ways you can take care of yourself so that you will be better able to care for your child.

❏ Complete routine physical and dental appointments that are due in the near future.

❏ Refill necessary prescriptions. Arrange to have prescriptions refilled away from home if needed.

❏ If you are under a physician's or therapist's care, discuss the care plan that you will follow while away. Arrange, if necessary, for medical or psychological care away from home.

Siblings

❏ Talk with other children about what will happen within the family while their brother or sister is going through a BMT. It is important to be honest, using words and concepts that your children can understand.

❏ Reassure children that you love them and that you will make plans for all family members so everyone will be taken care of. If children are staying at home, talk with them about who will be taking care of them.

❏ Discuss if there will be planned visits to the transplant center.

❏ If other children are coming along, talk with them about who will take care of them. Prepare siblings for the fact that parents may be taking turns caring for them along with caring for the patient.

Donor Sibling

❏ If a sibling is the donor, talk with the child honestly about his or her role as a donor, using words that he or she can understand.

❏ Explain what the schedule will be like, who will be with the child, and how he or she will be cared for.

❏ If the child is curious, inform him or her that the stem cells that are harvested from his or her body will replenish themselves.

❏ Talk about how his or her marrow or stem cells will help the brother or sister. You may want to explain the extent of his or her involvement in the donation and transplant process, as well as what will happen to the patient during recovery.

❏ If you want help talking with your child, ask your social worker or child family life specialist at your local hospital.

School

❑ Talk with your child's teacher(s) and principal about the transplant and how you can keep your child connected with the school, both academically and socially.

❑ Bring your child's schoolbooks and assignments along.

❑ Bring teacher and school contact information along.

❑ Depending on your circumstances, you may be able to enroll the patient and siblings in school programs near the transplant center. School enrollment may be available at the hospital, Ronald McDonald House, or in the community.

Faith/Spirituality

❑ If you have a faith community or place of worship, consider telling your faith leader and community where you will be. Perhaps establish a plan of communication (e-mail, cards, visits, telephone tree updates, etc.).

❑ Before coming to the transplant center, if you desire, ask your faith leader and community to offer special prayers, healing and annointing services, and other healing rituals for your child and family.

❑ Provide the time and opportunity to talk with your child and family about what each of you believes. Consider talking about what gives you comfort and strength as you and your family prepare for your child's transplant.

❑ You might consider bringing along sacred texts, prayers, prayer books, faith symbols (such as a rosary, prayer rug, cross, or Star of David), devotional and inspirational literature, music (CDs and tapes), faith-related videos, or other resources you may find helpful during the medical treatment.

Accommodations

❑ Make arrangements early for your housing and travel needs.

Financial

❑ Check with your insurance case manager to learn if there is coverage for housing, travel, and medical expenses related to your child's transplant.

❑ If you receive medical assistance, talk with your caseworker about financial assistance for travel, housing, and meals for the patient and caregiver.

❑ You may consider participating in fundraising activities for uncovered expenses related to your child's transplant. If you have applied for medical assistance or Supplemental Security Income (SSI), talk to your caseworker or social worker about how to protect any money raised so that it does not affect your child's eligibility for assistance.

Family and Friends

❑ Consider having a family photograph taken. Bring a copy along and leave a copy with any family members (such as siblings) remaining at home.

❑ Participate in a send-off gathering with family and friends.

❑ If friends and family want to know how they can help or what they can send, consider long-distance calling cards, snacks, meal certificates, notes of caring and encouragement, videos of family and friends, and items that you and your child might enjoy.

Communication

❏ Plan for how you will stay in touch with family members and friends back home.

❏ Bring long-distance calling cards.

❏ Bring telephone numbers, addresses, and e-mail addresses.

❏ Consider using videotapes or audiotapes to maintain contact with separated siblings and parents.

Packing List

❏ Make your own packing list as you think of things you want to bring.

❏ Bring items that will give comfort to your child and you.

❏ Bring loose clothing for your child, including shirts and pajamas that button in the front. This will provide easy access to his or her central venous catheter.

❏ Consider bringing some photos that are meaningful and uplifting.

❏ Refer to the packing list in the BMT information packet provided by your social worker.

Adapted from "Preparation Checklist for Pediatric Patients: Blood and Marrow Transplant Program at Fairview-University Medical Center," developed by Caroline Gale, LICSW; Doris Knettel, LICSW; Stacy Stickney Ferguson, LICSW; Janet Ziegler, LICSW; University of Minnesota Medical Center, Fairview, BMT Social Workers; and Kate Montgomery, LICSW, at the Office of Patient Advocacy at the National Marrow Donor Program.

APPENDIX C

GETTING READY TO LEAVE THE TRANSPLANT CENTER: FREQUENTLY ASKED QUESTIONS

After your transplant, you will receive information about when to call the doctor to report a fever, how to take medications, and whom to call for emergencies. You will see your transplant center doctor often while your new stem cells are growing.

The next major step is leaving the transplant center and returning to your primary care doctor. For many people, the transplant center is far from home. What information should you take with you when you leave? We hope the following questions and general guidelines will help you prepare for this transition.

This Q & A list contains only general guidelines. Your transplant center may have more specific guidelines for you to follow. Check with your transplant doctor or nurse coordinator for specifics regarding your situation.

Continuing Medical Care

What medical information has been sent to my primary care doctor? Does he or she know whom to call with questions about my transplant?

The transplant doctor will generally send a letter to your primary care doctor with a summary of your transplant course. Some transplant doctors will also call. Your primary care doctor will be given information on how to contact the transplant team. He or she will also be told what symptoms to look for, such as those for graft-versus-host disease (GVHD). Your medical record does not need to be sent.

What information should I carry with me?

You may ask for copies of the most recent notes and test results to bring to your primary care doctor. You should always have a list of your current medications and doses with you. Keep basic records for yourself for your future medical care.

When should I or my primary care doctor call the transplant doctor for advice? What symptoms are serious enough that I would have to go back to the transplant center for more follow-up care or tests?

You or your doctor can call the transplant nurse coordinator any time for advice. You should talk to your transplant doctor or nurse if you develop GVHD or if your GVHD symptoms get worse. Your transplant team may recommend a change in treatment.

What are the warning signs of chronic GVHD?

Sores in the mouth and pain or grittiness in the eyes may be signs of GVHD. Other signs include skin rash, nausea/vomiting, trouble swallowing, shortness of breath, persistent dry cough, numbness, tingling, and weakness.

Should I wear an ID bracelet to let people know I have had a BMT and might need special care?

An ID bracelet is optional, but it is a good idea. The information would tell people that you have had a BMT and that you should only receive irradiated blood products.

I still need to have blood products and antibiotics regularly. Who will arrange this for me?

Your BMT nurse or doctor will communicate directly with your primary care doctor and an appointment will be scheduled as soon as possible when you return home. If needed, a home care nursing visit may be arranged.

Before Going Home (When You Live in a Different Town)

What other issues should I think about before leaving the transplant center?

If you rented an apartment during your transplant stay, you may need to take care of several chores before you leave. Do you need to cancel any utility services in your name? Have you told your apartment management that you are leaving? Have you forwarded your mail?

There are many people that I have formed friendships with during the past several months. How do I stay in touch?

Say your good-byes to important people with whom you have connected during the past months. You may want to exchange addresses with other families that you have come to know.

Preparing the Home Environment

How do I need to prepare my home?

Keeping the home clean is important. You should not do the dusting or vacuuming or be in the room when dust is in the air. Do not have any remodeling work done on your home at this time.

Can I still care for my pets?

It's okay to be around pets that you had before your transplant. Check with your doctor about birds or reptiles, though. Let others do pet care such as grooming or waste removal. It is not a good idea to bring home a new pet during the first year after transplant.

Educating Visitors

How do I teach people what they need to do, such as hand washing, before they come to visit?

Think about how you want to communicate to your friends and family about the importance of precautions. Explain to friends and family that your doctor gave rules for your protection. This may help them understand that hand washing is the best way to keep infections from spreading.

How long do I enforce hand washing rules?

Good hand washing should be maintained at all times, especially before preparing food, after going to the bathroom, and after playing with pets.

Should there be a limit to the number of people in the room when we are at home?

Smaller groups are better if your white blood cell counts are low or if you are being treated for GVHD and receiving immunotherapy.

When should visitors or family members wear masks in the house?

Generally, masks are not worn at home. Visitors who are sick are discouraged from visiting. Family members should use proper hand-washing procedures.

Getting Back to Normal

When does life return to normal?

When you return home, life doesn't return to normal right away. Just as life changed when you got sick, it will change again as you become stronger. You'll gradually want to start taking on the tasks you did before. It's important to continue to talk about changes with your family and friends.

What types of social activities do I need to stay away from for the next few months? When can I get back to more normal social activities?

Your immune system is still recovering during the first year after an allogeneic stem cell transplant. When your white blood cell count is low (absolute neutrophil count less than 1000) or you are taking medicine that suppresses your immune system, you should stay away from enclosed, crowded places. If you are planning to eat out or go to a movie, choose a time when it is not busy.

When may I resume sexual activity?

While you are healing, your interest in sexual activity may be low due to lack of energy and not feeling well. Resuming sexual activity is a normal part of recovery, but each person must take it at his or her own pace. If you have questions or worries, you should discuss them with your doctor or nurse. There are many ways to remain close to your partner, such as holding each other, sitting close, holding hands, and spending time together doing things you both enjoy. The American Cancer Society offers information for men and women that focuses on sexuality and cancer.

When will my energy level improve? When will my counts be more in the normal range? How do I tell the difference between my physical recovery from the transplant and a new problem?

People get their energy back at different times, some sooner than others. It's normal to take lots of naps. Patience is needed, as your energy will return slowly. If you are taking medication for GVHD, your immune system and energy level will not recover as quickly. Any major energy level change should be reported to your doctor. It is normal to feel good one day and overdo activity, making you tired the next day. Try to save your energy by pacing yourself with moderate amounts of activity.

Back to Work

When may I go back to work? What should I tell my employer about how long I will be out on disability?

Ask your doctor about the estimated length of your disability. You may qualify for Social Security Disability Insurance (SSDI) or Supplemental Security Income (SSI). Your human resources representative at work or the hospital social worker can help you understand how these programs may apply to your situation.

What are my rights concerning disability, and how long will I be able to keep my job and my insurance coverage?

Contact your employer regarding extended absence from work. Seek out your employee human resources representative to help you understand your benefits and responsibilities in order to qualify for extended disability and continuation of medical insurance.

When I am ready to return to work, what can I do if I feel I'm being discriminated against based on my medical history?

Under federal law and many state laws, an employer cannot treat you differently than other workers based on a medical diagnosis if you are qualified for the job. To understand your rights, contact The National Coalition for Cancer Survivorship for information and publications.

Back to School

When can a child return to school following a BMT?

Children may return to school from six months to a year after transplant. It depends on the recovery of your child's immune system and physical strength. Until your child returns to school, you can make plans with the school (an Individual Education Plan) to keep your child involved in his or her schoolwork. Your child may be eligible for home tutoring and other programs that meet his or her educational needs. When it is time to go back to school, contact your hospital social worker, nurse, or school counselor for videos, written materials, and ideas to make going back to school easier for your child.

Exercising

How much exercise is safe? Can I go swimming? Horseback riding? Skiing? If not now, when?

Exercise should be gentle and in moderation. When your platelets are low, falls can result in serious bleeding. Walking is one of the best forms of exercise at this time. Consult your doctor before resuming rigorous exercise. You can't swim until your central venous catheter is removed and the site has healed; swimming pools can be an easy place to pick up infections. Postpone strenuous activities for several months until your doctor determines that you are ready.

When can I work in the garden or yard?

Wait six months to one year before digging in the dirt or mowing the lawn. If you have GVHD, ask your physician when you can begin working in your yard or garden. Wear your mask on windy days when there may be dust or dirt in the air.

Dealing with Emotions and Finding Support

What types of support will I need when I return home?

When you first get home, you may need a support network, but those you have counted on in the past may not know this. There will still be times when you cannot be alone or when you will need assistance during the day. There will still be many doctor appointments and transportation needs. The positive side is that home is where your family and friends are located. It's time to get back in touch and ask for help.

Where can I find a support group to fit my needs?

Ask for referrals from social workers, your local American Cancer Society, your local Leukemia and Lymphoma Society, or Cancer Care. Talk honestly with family and friends to help them understand the types of support that you find helpful.

What kind of support is available for caregivers?

Look for caregiver support groups. While these groups may focus on a variety of caregiver issues, most caregivers will find they have many common concerns.

How can I work through the changes in my physical appearance?

Your body may go through many changes following transplant. These may include hair loss, weight gain or loss, a puffy face due to steroids, and changes in skin condition from GVHD. You may have scars from medical procedures such as placement of your central venous catheter. Most of these changes are temporary. A support group or therapist could help you adjust to any changes in your physical appearance.

Sometimes it feels like I've been through a war. How do I process all that I've been through?

This may be the time to talk through your experience with a therapist. Different issues may come up at different times, even one year or several years after the transplant.

I am glad to leave the transplant center and be through with this part of treatment, but I am very scared about what's going to happen next. Who can I talk to? Do others feel the same way? Why does everyone expect me to be happy?

You may find that you have a need to talk with others in similar situations. There are organizations that can connect you with other transplant survivors by phone or e-mail. Some people find the need to talk to a therapist who has treated post-traumatic stress disorder or who has worked with people who have health-related trauma.

Talking with Family

What concerns might my family have when I return home?

Returning home is a happy time, but problems that existed before the transplant may now resurface. Communication is more important than ever. Some family members will want everything to return to the way it was before transplant, but recovery takes time.

Are children going to have specific concerns?

Children who have had alternate caregivers may need time to adjust to being together again as a family. Children may need to test rules and may show anger. Trust between parent and child may need to be rebuilt. Siblings can also experience adjustment issues as the family is reunited. Be patient and realize that it will take some time to settle into the new routine.

Traveling

When should I avoid travel by plane? Is this dependent on my platelet or white blood cell counts?

Many people plan to return to their homes by airplane. Air travel is not restricted if your blood counts are low.

Is it safe for me to drive?

Some medications may cause drowsiness or affect concentration and reflexes; check with your doctor before driving a car. You may be a passenger in a car.

Finding Financial Information

If my work disability is coming to an end, are there other programs that provide income?

The federal government has two income insurance programs available for adults: Social Security Disability Insurance (SSDI) and Supplemental Security Income (SSI). Eligibility is based on a determination by your doctor that your disability will last one year or longer. SSDI is based on money you have paid into social security through payroll tax. SSI is a program for people (including children under eighteen) who are disabled and have limited incomes and resources. You may already qualify to start receiving benefits based on your income or date of disability. Contact your local social security office as soon as possible to apply. If you are covered under your employer's disability plan (short- or long-term), the employer will assist you in deciding when to apply. Those who qualify for SSI (based on meeting minimum income requirements) may also be eligible for Medicaid, which can help cover medical costs.

I'm a veteran. Do I qualify for additional income?

Veterans should contact their local veterans administration office to inquire if they are eligible for any programs based on their service record and disability.

Thinking about Long-term Effects

What are the long-term effects of a BMT?

Long-term effects may include possible disease relapse, secondary malignancy (cancer), cataracts, infertility, ovarian failure, short-term memory loss, and numbness or tingling of the feet or hands. Some of these might not surface until years after your transplant. Make sure you tell your doctor if you have any of these effects.

Do precautions need to be taken when outdoors during the day?

If you will be outdoors at all in bright or hazy sun, always wear sunscreen on all exposed skin. Use SPF 30 or higher to prevent sunburn or activation of GVHD.

How can I deal with dry eyes and dry mouth?

Use artificial tears (eyedrops) and suck on hard candy for dry mouth. Drink plenty of fluids. Your doctor may have additional suggestions.

What are some of the signs of depression? I have heard that some people suffer from post-traumatic stress syndrome. How can I recognize if I have a serious emotional problem?

Many of the signs of depression are similar to symptoms of medical problems, such as difficulty eating or irregular sleep patterns. It is always good to first check with your doctor to rule out any physical problems associated with your treatment. If you are unable to concentrate, feel overly emotional or as though you lack emotions, and have been feeling unhappy for several weeks, you may need to consult a therapist or psychiatrist to see if you are suffering from depression or a related disorder. There are medical treatments to help, and talking with a therapist can assist your recovery.

What should I know about the long-term effects of transplant on children?

If transplant occurs before puberty, a child may not reach sexual maturity. If a BMT occurs prior to adolescence, there may be concerns about achieving normal growth or experiencing difficulty in school. There are many interventions that can assist parents in helping their children manage these effects. Starting early is important in dealing with these concerns. (Recommended reading: *Childhood Cancer Survivors: A Practical Guide to Your Future* by Nancy Keene, Wendy Hobbie, and Kathy Ruccione.)

Sometimes it's difficult to be a transplant survivor. What can I do with the experience I've gained?

Many patients, caregivers, and loved ones want to do something with the hard-won knowledge they've gained from their experiences. And many organizations look to transplant survivors to share their experiences with others who are just starting out. For more information, contact your hospital social worker or any of the organizations listed in the Resources section for ideas on how to share your transplant journey with others.

This information was adapted from materials developed by Kate Montgomery, LICSW, at the Office of Patient Advocacy at the National Marrow Donor Program in collaboration with University of Minnesota Medical Center, Fairview, BMT Social Workers, Caroline Gale, LICSW, Doris Knettel, LICSW, Stacy Stickney Ferguson, LICSW, and Janet Ziegler, LICSW.

GLOSSARY

Absolute neutrophil count—the number of neutrophils, white blood cells that are the primary defense for fighting infection from bacteria and yeast.

Allogeneic transplant—a transplant in which stem cells are donated from a related or unrelated donor whose tissue is a close match to that of the person having the transplant.

Antibiotic—a drug used to fight infections.

Antigens—proteins in the body that are recognized by the immune system and can produce an immune response.

Apheresis—a procedure to collect peripheral blood cells by drawing blood and circulating it through a machine that removes the stem cells and returns the remaining blood cells to the person.

Autologous transplant—a transplant using the patient's own stem cells.

Biopsy—the removal of a sample of body tissue to examine it for signs of disease.

Bone marrow—spongy tissue inside the bones where all blood cells are produced.

Bone marrow aspiration—a procedure used to obtain bone marrow to examine for disease or engraftment.

Bone marrow collection or harvest—surgical procedure for obtaining bone marrow for transplantation.

Bone marrow transplant—a procedure used to treat some cancers and other diseases. After high-dose chemotherapy and radiation, damaged bone marrow is replaced with new bone marrow cells.

Central venous catheter—a small, long, flexible plastic tube, usually inserted into a vein in the neck or chest. Used to administer medications, fluids, and nutrition and for collecting stem cells. Also referred to as a CVC or RAC (right atrial catheter).

Chemotherapy—treatment with one or more anticancer drugs to stop or slow the growth of cancer cells.

Colony-stimulating factors—proteins that stimulate the production and growth of blood cells; see *Growth factors*.

Conditioning or preparative treatment—high-dose chemotherapy and/or radiation given to kill cancer cells and suppress the immune system before a BMT.

Cultures—body tissue, blood, or body fluid obtained to test for infection.

Echocardiogram (ECHO)—a test used to visualize abnormal heart motion.

Electrocardiogram (ECG or EKG)—a test that measures electrical currents in the heart to detect irregularities or heart injury.

Engraftment—the process in which transplanted stem cells begin to grow in the bone marrow and manufacture new blood cells.

Erythrocytes—see *Red blood cells*.

Graft—the new stem cells that are transplanted and begin to grow in the recipient's bone marrow after the transplant.

Graft failure—a complication after BMT in which the transplanted stem cells do not grow in the recipient's bone marrow and thus do not produce new blood cells.

Graft-versus-host disease (GVHD)—a complication after BMT in which the transplanted stem cells cause the recipient's new immune system to attack his or her own body cells and tissue.

Growth factors—medications that increase the number of stem cells in the blood by stimulating the production and growth of blood cells.

Hematopoietic stem cells—"parent cells" of all blood cells. Stem cells divide into red blood cells, white blood cells, and platelets.

Hemoglobin—molecules in red blood cells that carry oxygen.

Human leukocyte antigen (HLA) typing—a way to identify proteins (antigens) on the surface of white blood cells that serve as unique markers distinguishing one person from another; also called *tissue typing*.

Immune system—the organs and cells in the body that fight infection and disease.

IV—abbreviation for *intravenous* or *intravenously,* meaning into or within a vein.

Leukapheresis—a procedure to collect the white blood cell and stem cell portion of the blood. See also *Apheresis.*

Leukocytes—see *White blood cells.*

Lumbar puncture—see *Spinal tap.*

Lymphocytes—white blood cells that help protect the body against viral infections.

Mobilization—using growth factor drugs and/or chemotherapy to move stem cells from the bone marrow into the bloodstream for collection.

Neutrophils—white blood cells that help protect the body against bacterial and yeast infections.

Peripheral blood stem cells—stem cells that circulate in the blood.

Peripheral blood stem cell donation—having stem cells removed from blood through a process called *apheresis*, which takes the stem cells out of the blood and returns the remaining blood back to the donor.

Peripheral blood stem cell transplant—a procedure used to treat advanced cancer and other diseases; stem cells are removed from the blood and transplanted, or reinfused, into the patient.

Platelet—blood cells that make the blood clot.

Pre-transplant evaluation—a medical examination before BMT; also called *workup*.

Priming chemotherapy—chemotherapy given to increase the number of stem cells in the blood.

Radiation—treatment to destroy cancer cells and immune system using high-energy rays from X-rays, electron beams, or radioisotopes.

Red blood cells—cells that carry oxygen from the lungs to all parts of the body; also called *erythrocytes*.

Spinal tap (LP, or lumbar puncture)—a procedure used to obtain spinal fluid. A small needle is inserted between two vertebrae into the spinal canal. Fluid is then withdrawn and examined for disease or infection.

Stem cells—"parent" cells that divide and form the cells that make up the blood and immune system.

Stem cell collection, harvest, or retrieval—the process of removing stem cells from blood; see also *Apheresis* and *Leukapheresis*.

T cells (or T lymphocytes)—white blood cells that tell the body to attack foreign cells, which could cause infections.

Tissue typing—see *Human leukocyte antigen (HLA) typing*.

Total parenteral nutrition (TPN)—nutrition provided directly into the bloodstream.

White blood cells—blood cells that fight infection; also called *leukocytes*.

Workup—see *Pre-transplant evaluation*.

Resources

BONE MARROW AND STEM CELL TRANSPLANT

American Bone Marrow Donor Registry

P.O. Box 8841
Mandeville, LA 70470-8841
(800) 745-2452
http://www.abmdr.org

American Cancer Society

1599 Clifton Road NE
Atlanta, GA 30329
(404) 320-3333
(800) 227-2345
http://cancer.org

American Society of Blood and Marrow Transplant (ASBMT)

85 W. Algonquin Road, Suite 550
Arlington Heights, IL 60005
(847) 427-0224
http://www.asbmt.org

Blood and Marrow Transplant Information Network

2900 Skokie Valley Road, Suite B
Highland Park, IL 60035
(847) 433-3313
(888) 597-7674
http://www.bmtinfonet.org

The Blood and Marrow Transplant Program at the University of Minnesota Medical Center, Fairview

420 Delaware Street SE, MMC 803
Minneapolis, MN 55455
(612) 273-2800
(888) 601-0787
(800) 328-5576 [accommodations]
http://www.fairviewbmt.org
http://www.peds.umn.edu/Centers/BMT

Cancer Care

275 7th Avenue
New York, NY 10001
(800) 813-4673
http://www.cancercare.org

Cancer Information Service/ National Cancer Institute (CIS/NCI)

6116 Executive Boulevard, MSC 8322
Room 3036A
Bethesda, MD 20892
(800) 4-CANCER [422-6237]
http://www.cancer.gov

Candlelighters Childhood Cancer Foundation

P.O. Box 498
Kensington, MD 20895
(800) 366-2223
http://www.candlelighters.org

Caring Bridge

4607 Beacon Hill, Suite 200
Eagan, MN 55122-2702
(651) 452-7940
http://www.caringbridge.org

Coping with Cancer Magazine

P.O. Box 682268
Franklin, TN 37068
(615) 790-2400
http://www.copingmag.com

International Bone Marrow Transplant Registry/Autologous Blood and Marrow Transplant Registry

IBMTR/ABMTR Statistical Center
Health Policy Institute, Medical College of Wisconsin
8701 Watertown Plank Road, P.O. Box 26509
Milwaukee, WI 53226
(414) 456-8325
http://www.ibmtr.org

Kids Konnected

27071 Cabot Road, Suite 102
Laguna Hills, CA 92653
(800) 899-2866
http://www.kidskonnected.org

Leukemia and Lymphoma Society

1311 Mamaroneck Avenue
White Plains, NY 10605
http://www.leukemia-lymphoma.org

Lymphoma Research Foundation

111 Broadway, 19th Floor
New York, NY 10006
(800) 235-6848
http://www.lymphoma.org

National Association of Hospital Hospitality Houses

P.O. Box 18087
Ashville, NC 28814-0087
(800) 542-9730
http://www.nahhh.org

National Bone Marrow Transplant Link

20411 W. 12 Mile Road, Suite 108
Southfield, MI 48076
(248) 358-1886
(800) 546-5268
http://www.comnet.org/nbmtlink

National Children's Cancer Society

115 Locust, Suite 600
St. Louis, MO 63101
(800) 352-6459
http://www.children-cancer.org

National Coalition for Cancer Survivorship

1010 Wayne Avenue, Suite 770
Silver Spring, MD 20910
(301) 650-9127
http://www.canceradvocacy.org

National Family Caregivers Association

10400 Connecticut Avenue, Suite 500
Kensington, MD 20895
(800) 896-3650
http://www.nfcacares.org

National Marrow Donor Program

3001 Broadway Street NE, Suite 500
Minneapolis, MN 55413-1753
(800) 627-7692
http://www.marrow.org

Oncology Nursing Society

125 Enterprise Drive
Pittsburgh, PA 15275
(866) 257-4667
http://www.ons.org

Starbright Foundation

11835 W. Olympic Boulevard, Suite 500
Los Angeles, CA 90064
(310) 479-1212
(800) 315-2580
http://www.starbright.org

The Wellness Community

919 18th Street NW, #LL54
Washington, DC 20006
(202) 659-9709
(888) 793-9355
http://www.thewellnesscommunity.org

INFERTILITY

American Society for Reproductive Medicine

1209 Montgomery Highway
Birmingham, AL 35216-2809
(205) 978-5000
http://www.asrm.org

Genetics and In Vitro Fertilization Institute

3020 Javier Road
Fairfax, VA 22031
(800) 552-4363
http://www.givf.com

Resolve: The National Fertility Association

1310 Broadway
Somerville, MA 02144
(888) 623-0744
http://www.resolve.org

INSURANCE AND FINANCIAL ASSISTANCE

Association of Community Cancer Centers

11600 Nebel Street, #201
Rockville, MD 20852
(301) 984-9496
http://www.accc-cancer.org

Bone Marrow Foundation

337 East 88th Street, Suite 1B
New York, NY 10128
(212) 838-3029
(800) 365-1336
http://www.bonemarrow.org

Health Insurance Association of America

1201 F Street NW, Suite 500
Washington, DC 20004
(202) 824-1600
http://www.hiaa.org

The Marrow Foundation

400 Seventh Street NW, Suite 206
Washington, DC 20004
(202) 638-6601
(800) 627-7692
http://www.themarrowfoundation.org

National Foundation for Transplants

1102 Brookfield, Suite 200
Memphis, TN 38119
(800) 489-3863
http://www.transplants.org

National Marrow Donor Program

Office of Patient Advocacy
3001 Broadway Street NE, Suite 500
Minneapolis, MN 55413-1753
(888) 999-6743
http://www.marrow.org

National Transplant Assistance Fund

3475 West Chester Pike, Suite 230
Newtown Square, PA 19073
(800) 642-8399
http://www.transplantfund.org

Patient Advocacy Coalition

777 E. Girard Avenue
Englewood, CO 80113
(303) 744-7667
http://www.patientadvocacy.net

Patient Advocate Foundation

700 Thimble Shoals Boulevard, Suite 200
Newport News, VA 23606
(800) 532-5274
http://www.patientadvocate.org

Social Security Administration

(800) 772-1213
http://www.ssa.gov

TRANSPORTATION SUPPORT

Angel Flight America

National Office
P.O. Box 17467
Memphis, TN 38187
(877) 621-7177
http://www.airlifeline.org

Corporate Angel Network Inc.

Westchester County Airport
1 Loop Road
White Plains, NY 10604
(866) 328-1313
http://www.corpangelnetwork.org

National Patient Air Transport Helpline

4620 Haygood Road, Suite 1
Virginia Beach, VA 23455
(800) 296-1217
http://www.patienttravel.org

INDEX

bowel habits, changes in, 34, 36, 39, 44-45, 47, 54-55, 66, 73-74
breathing difficulties, 3, 37, 55-56, 66, 84, 128
breathing exercises, 110
bronchiolitis obliterans, 84
bronchitis, 56, 84

caffeine, 71, 74, 158
calorie counts, 69, 78
calorie intake, 45, 69-70, 78
cancer, 2, 4, 8, 33, 52, 83, 86, 90, 114, 131, 133-134, 137-138, 142, 144, 147-151, 153. See also specific types.
candida, 48. See also yeast.
carbohydrates, 73
caregiving, 9, 13-14, 61, 99, 102-103, 134
case manager, transplant. See insurance representative.
cataracts, 84, 137
central venous catheter (CVC), 5-6, 13, 23, 32, 34, 36, 126, 135, 142; 60, 103, 133; and infections, 46, 48
chaplains, 42, 91, 97, 104, 118, 121
chemotherapy, 34; effects on children, 35, 84-86; priming, 31, 144; side effects of, 34-35, 83, 92
chickenpox, 50, 57, 67
child family life (CFL) specialists, 42, 114, 121
children, 16-18, 23, 26, 36, 42, 54, 60, 63, 84-86, 90, 103, 105, 114, 121, 123, 133, 136, 138, 148, 150; as stem cell donors, 6, 27, 29-30, 119, 123; of BMT patients, 99, 104-105, 109, 114, 116-117, 121-126, 133. See also pediatric patients.
chills, 36-37, 48, 65

church. See faith community.
clinical trials. See research studies.
COBRA, 116
colds, 47, 67
cold sores, 49
colony-stimulating factor. See growth factor medications.
communication, 82, 94, 103-104, 114, 124, 126, 129-130, 135
complications, 22, 30, 34, 40-41, 43, 45, 47, 49-50, 52-53, 55, 90, 143; and allogeneic transplants, 26, 39-41, 51, 53, 60. See also specific complications
conditioning therapy, 33
consent forms, 22-23
constipation, 73
consultations, 11, 22
copays, 15
coughing, 55, 65, 128
CT scan, 22, 33
cytomegalovirus (CMV), 49

dairy products, 74. See also lactose intolerance.
day zero, 36
death, 17, 91, 93, 95-96, 98, 106
deliberate relaxation, 42
denial, 89, 94
dental floss, 41
depression, 18, 83, 89-90, 92-93, 101, 108-110, 138
diagnosis, 11, 56, 133
dialysis, 18
diarrhea, 34, 36, 39, 45, 47, 54-55, 66, 73-74; causes of, 44-45; solutions for, 73-74
dietitian, 45, 68, 70, 73-74, 78
digestive tract, 48, 56, 70; biopsy, 54
dirt, working in, 134

disability, 15, 17-18, 115-118, 132, 136-137; and discrimination, 117, 133
Disability Determination Services, 17
discharge from hospital, 2, 30, 40, 47, 59-62, 66, 69-70, 78, 92, 103, 113, 129
distraction from pain, 42
donors, 27-28, 89, 98, 145, 151; matching, 2, 6-7, 25-28, 52, 141; related, 5-6, 26-28, 51, 141; unrelated, 2, 5-6, 26-27, 51, 141
donor registries, 27, 147
driving, 13, 30, 61, 85, 102, 136, 151
dry mouth, 137; solutions for, 72
dusting, 49, 130, 134

eating problems, 70-72, 76, 138. See also specific problems.
echocardiogram (MUGA), 22, 142
electrocardiogram (ECG or EKG), 22, 28, 142
electrolytes, 69
emergency assistance, 13, 103, 117, 127
emotional preparation, 9, 12, 18-19, 102
emotional support, 14, 52, 97, 99, 102-105, 134
employee assistance programs, 116
employer, 116-117, 122, 132-133, 137
endoscope, 54
endurance, 62
energy level, 35, 80, 132
engraftment, 25, 37-38, 142
estate planning, 116
Ewing's sarcoma, 8
exercise, 42, 59, 69, 71, 73,